<u>Becoming A Personal Trainer</u>

Connect With Clients, Grow Your Business, and Keep Your F***ing Sanity

BECOMING A PERSONAL TRAINER

First edition. October 18, 2024.

Copyright © 2024 Mia Lazarewicz.

ISBN: 979-8227271167

Written by Mia Lazarewicz.

Table of Contents

This book is dedicated to all of my clients over the years,

who taught me everything I know about this work.

Chapter One: Introduction

I nearly quit my job when The Author/Filmmaker—a woman who would leave me voicemails identifying herself by her profession rather than her name—asked me to take off my pants at the beginning of our session. "If you cared about your clients at all, you would do this for me," she said. We were in the middle of the gym floor, and she was edging closer, like a rattlesnake slithering towards its cornered prey.

"I'm...not going to loan you my pants," I said, hesitantly. It's hard to imagine that I wasn't **absolutely** certain that I would not be removing my pants and working for an hour in my underwear, but she was terrifying. In the moment, I was absolutely not certain of that.

"Just give me your pants."

"No."

"Well, at least give me your sneakers."

"No."

"I cannot BELIEVE that you are willing to jeopardize my LIFE just because you don't want to loan your stuff out for one hour. It's so SELFISH. Put a towel around your waist and give me your pants."

"I will not. I'm sorry." Proud of myself for this brave reply in the face of being at work in a personal training jacket, bath towel, and bare feet.

"Fine. Then I just have to work out in my tights. If I slip and fall, it's your fault and I WILL pursue damages."

She disappeared down into the locker room and re-emerged, to my intense delight, as promised, in a long-sleeve tee-shirt and sheer black tights. I'm talking sheer. The next forty minutes were like being in a sideshow, where gym members would do double-takes as they passed by The Pantsless Woman. I tried to be professional, but it was really fucking funny. One of those times where you're looking around in disbelief, wondering how you ended up in that specific moment in time and space.

I didn't quit that day, or any other day, even though every session with her was worthy of my leaving the field forever. She used to enter our gym like Miranda Priestly: dumping her coat, purse, and keys across the front desk, purring, "Can you hold my BMW keys," to our front desk guy as she breezed by, twenty minutes late. She once was extra late, and then screamed at me for not giving her a wake-up call.

"I'm *always* on really important phone calls with Europe. I can't be expected to keep a normal schedule when my work is so important. Frankly, I don't think it's too much to ask that you could give me a call before each session." What I said is that I wasn't her butler, but what I wanted to say was "Fuuuuuuuckkkkk youuuuuuuuuuuuuuuuu."

I trained her for a year before I finally had enough clients to afford getting rid of her. I sent her an email gently saying that I wouldn't be renewing our sessions together and would be happy to set her up with another trainer. (I intended to give her to my asshole coworker. I'd never inflict her on someone I liked.) She wrote a reply that started with, "Hi Mia, thanks so much for understanding how unsatisfactory your training has been." It still makes me laugh today. I was also told that she mailed an iconic three-page letter about me to our corporate offices in Colorado, but, in one of the great disappointments of my life, I never got to see it.

Personal training is a unique and fantastic career. There will be assholes, of course, because it's a service job. All service jobs come with hairy assholes. They are hairier than you could have ever imagined, and they are assholey.

But they are only a small negative of the personal training equation, and nearly all the rest of the coefficients are positive. There are so many excellent reasons to become a personal trainer. Help people! Contribute to public health! New friends! Good money! Free gym membership! Make your own hours! Coworkers with similar interests! Wear sweatpants all day! Make a living by telling people what to do! (A bossy child's dream.) All this for the price of a certificate that runs a couple hundred bucks. The return on the personal training career investment is insane.

But there are some pitfalls to the field, and all of the worst ones come right in the beginning. If you can't navigate the unpleasant starting points, you won't be able to enjoy all the good stuff that comes later (AKA writing off your massive sneaker collection as a work expense).

This book will show you all the pitfalls I never knew about when I was a baby trainer (and the coping mechanisms to handle them), along with the wonderful job perks you probably never realized were part of the gig (World Series tickets, free shoes, a career which is a fantastic conversation starter, and stories about your client wanting you to work on the gym floor in your underwear).

In the beginning, you're not gonna make any money and you're not gonna know what you're doing and you're gonna have to train a few dickheads while you build up your clientele. But if you follow my advice, you'll be able to overcome all of these problems and more. And it'll be worth it, because you'll be teaching people how to understand and respect the hell out of their own bodies. And not respect in a *Do you want to know the circumference of my biceps?* kind of way, but in a *I want to be mountain climbing for my 90th birthday* kind of way.

Everyone thinks that personal trainers are here to help people become jacked and hot, but that's a small part of what we do. We're really in it for the longterm effects. Huge, sexy, biceps are a dream but they're not gonna hold up to scrutiny as your clients age. What *does* hold up to scrutiny? Intelligent cardio program design, full-body strength training, understanding injuries, mobility work, and walking as much as humanly possible.

Now, if you build them some gorgeous biceps on top of that? Then you have truly given your clients everything.

Come with me to find out the pros and cons of training as a career, understanding the certification process, how to meet clients and run their first workouts, how to cultivate great relationships built on trust, how to comfortably sell expensive exercise, and even how to take this gym-based service knowledge and apply it to be great at any other service field. Plus, you want gym gossip? There's some real hot tea spilled throughout the book, including the influencers who make me rage, some shocking interactions with physical therapists, and my thoughts on the fitness industry at large. Believe me, they are not all good thoughts. In a lot of ways, the industry is a mess. For most fields, the public-facing parts are squeaky clean and it's only the private parts that are dirty. (Like your mom.) In health and wellness, the outside-facing parts are just as dirty as the inside. (Like your sister.) We'll talk about all of it, along with ways that you can help make it better.

One thing is for sure: one badass career lies in front of you. A career where you can leave the desk behind, leave computer screens behind, leave Chad from Marketing behind, leave the pointless grind of making someone else super rich, and help people literally change their lives.

Let's go.

Like so many people, I became a personal trainer because I didn't have any other job prospects. I am not sure what makes all of us go, *Hey! I like gyms and I have no other prospects! I should be a personal trainer,* but that's how most of us end up here. It's a classic interim job, sort of like ski bumming, where you intend to do it for a short time until you figure out something real to do with your life. I'm not sure what the specific draw to fitness is; it's not a very good interim job, which we'll talk more about later. And people have lots of other interests that don't usually lure them into jobs. I've never angled to work in a donut shop, cat café, or giant dildo store. I suspect we chose fitness because if we're getting paid to exercise, that essentially makes us professional athletes, which is phenomenal content for the Tinder bio.

Personal training never crossed my mind as a full-time job I might want to have. I was working nights as a cheerleading coach when I took a day job as a gym equipment cleaner in Cambridge, MA. I don't care about cleaning equipment but I do very much care about the free gym membership you get when you clean equipment. Perk #1 of being a personal trainer: you get all the fitness for free.

Everyone thinks they'd be amazing at dishing out their favorite locker room lifting secrets. Huge shout out to the guy I overheard telling his client to squat more because testosterone is made in the butt and squatting is how you release it to the rest of the body. (Spoiler alert: no. Also, can you imagine if we had to pump prime our butts like a piston in order to release hormones into the body? Like, hold on, attacking bear, I need my ass adrenaline.)

It is alluring, but most people will have a tough time making a real career at it. It's not tough because personal training is wicked hard. When I talk to my teacher friends, I'm embarrassed by how easy my work is in comparison. It's tough because it is the definition of a service job, and if you're not ready for a career in servitude, you're gonna be super, super unhappy as a personal trainer. My office-working friends can't fathom how I deal with people all day long. I tell them stories and they say, "Holy shit. I could never." That's why this book isn't about exercise. It's about people.

The service industry breaks down into three groups, and different types of people will do well in each of the three. If you want to work in service but the jobs you've tried haven't been it, it's possible you're just in the wrong branch. The personality and client-need requirements are different for each one. First you have the short-term professions of servitude: restaurant servers, bartenders, flight attendants, hospitality managers, house cleaners, front desk clerks, retail workers, tour guides, etc. I find these professions to be distinct in the service world because use of these professions is optional, and the quality of work is generally valued more than the personality of the worker. You can get your college tour, your food served, or your airplane snack from someone you like talking to, or someone you don't talk to at all. These jobs are elevated by a fantastic personality, but it's not required to be great at the job. The client wants good drinks first and foremost, and then it's just a bonus when the bartender is also super cool.

The fact that the clients and providers in these scenarios don't choose each other makes these jobs hard as hell. Every fucking asshole on the planet goes out to dinner and rides airplanes. I love working in my area of service, but I'd be the most miserable flight attendant you've ever met. I don't know how they do it. The minute Kristy and Kevin and their two shitty toddlers start throwing star pasta all over the seat while Arnold in the row behind them farts like he'll never find a toilet again, I'd be opening the escape hatch and launching myself down the slide and off the planet. Huge respect to this branch of service work.

Then you have the requisite service professions like lawyer, doctor, plumber, accountant, car mechanic, etc. These are the second part of the service economy, and they've got totally different personality and client-need requirements. These are vital services. People *need* their burst pipe fixed/accounts reconciled/cancer treated, and they need it done extremely well, so it's all about the skill. You don't need any kind of personality to be great at these professions, as anyone who's met a surgeon before knows.

But you do need a personality if people are going to pay optional money—and a lot of it—to spend time with you. They need to love you right from the start. This is where people in the third group shine. You're being hired for your disposition as much as for your work, so these people need physical skills *and* a great personality to succeed. Being great at the work isn't enough. People hire you by choice because they want to talk to you. They seek you out over others. They don't need you, they want you. This is massage therapy, manicurists, estheticians, wedding planners, therapists, hairdressers, real estate agents, and yes, personal trainers. You can be loud or quiet, gentle or aggressive, but if you cannot hold a good conversation, you will not be a successful personal trainer. So keep that in mind as you consider the field.

Lots of people who love to work out are terrible trainers. Anyone can teach a squat or a bicep curl. Strangely, that's not the defining successful characteristic of a trainer. So this book isn't about squats and bicep curls. This book is about service. And if you're not ready to provide a massive, all-consuming, sacrificial service to others, then you're not ready for a career as a personal trainer. I'm talking waking up at 4am or working til 10pm, skipping vacations, working holidays and weekends, spending hours writing training programs for people who won't do them, being treated like a servant, and being unafraid of sweaty, bloody, sobby clients, plus the occasional tit or testicle falling out of loose clothing.

What's in it for you, besides swass and nips? If you do it right, you'll be legitimately improving and ultimately changing people's lives. They will be able to hike mountains, pick up their child, and run marathons in part because of your work together. They will be happier in life because of your work together. On top of that, you can easily pull a six-figure salary (I crossed $100,000 annually in my third year in the field and never looked back); build an incredible network; make lifelong friendships; retain ultimate scheduling flexibility; gain a deep understanding of the human body; find opportunities for growth and entrepreneurship; receive plenty of cash tips at Christmas, get vacation homes being offered for use; get education in fields from neurology to nutrition to aging to biomechanics; and—the most crucial for me personally—never needing to work at a desk another day in your life.

Think you're ready to trade the deskicles for the testicles? Then read on.

Chapter Two: The Pros And Cons

The first things to consider about becoming a personal trainer are the pros and cons of the job. A lot of people love to exercise, so they think that being a trainer would be the most natural thing in the world. And it is, if you learn how to manage it well. But just because I love to argue with people doesn't make me a great lawyer. Just because I love spending every last dime I have on shopping doesn't mean a job in retail is right for me. You need to have more than a love of exercise to make it as a personal trainer. The good news is, I've done all of the fucking around for you, so that you can just read the finding out part.

Working as a personal trainer has some tremendous perks and some real big downfalls. Like all jobs, you'll need to decide if the perks outweigh the problems for you, and then—this part is critical—you need to let the problems go. I've known some excellent trainers over the years who could never make a career of it because they were too busy complaining about all the parts of the job they hated. I always felt their priorities were wrong. They were their own priority. And that's totally fine. But then you don't choose one of the serviest of all service jobs. When you work in service, you're not the priority.

You don't wanna work early, late, weekends, and holidays? I can tell you right now that service jobs aren't gonna be your jam. If that part isn't okay for you, you can stop reading now. Because this is key: People arrange for service work at the times when they themselves are not working. That means you work at 6am before they go to work. It means you work at 7pm when they're done with work. It means weekends and holidays. It means you need to be there to provide a service pretty much every time they want it. That makes your travel, vacations, and general free time difficult.

I can feel the Gen Z recoil from here. *Being a slave to your job is soooo millennial. What about self-care? You never need to be available all the time. It's giving menty b's.* They're not wrong, and have all the menty b's you want, but trust me on this one. People will not stay your client for long if you are not always available to work their sessions.

Imagine if you had a hairdresser you adored, but every time you tried to schedule her for a Saturday, she was gonna be away that weekend. She's only available Wednesday or Thursday mornings, when you're typically working. You finally have a free Wednesday, but she's gonna be in California that week. You could take time off from work on a Thursday but she's booked the next four Thursdays. Etc, etc. The effort to find a common time would only need to happen three or four times before you'd find a new hairdresser who could better accommodate your schedule. It's just too difficult.

The most important part: in this scenario, which is already so annoying, you're booking a service that you only get every couple months. People want to see their personal trainer one to four times a week. If you can't match their schedule—constantly—they will find another trainer who can.

So let's talk about scheduling first. Scheduling is one of the biggest cons AND one of the biggest pros of the job. But it is complicated and I think it's the thing that new trainers understand the least about what lies ahead.

Personal trainers get paid by the session, not by the hours they're physically at the gym. And if you don't have a lot of clients, on any given day you might have sessions at 7am, 10am, and 6pm. Assuming you can't get home easily in the interim, then you're at the gym for twelve hours, yet paid for three. If that sounds like it sucks, you're right.

So how do you ever manage to make a living before you get a ton of clients? There are two ways, and neither of them is great. The first way is floor hours. Most gyms offer them, which are minimum-wage hours, usually part-time, and they're meant for you to be cleaning equipment, offering members towels, running tables like blood pressure screenings or balance testing, and generally trying to drum up more business. These are intended to be phased out as you pick up clients. The gym doesn't want to pay you for wandering around, they want you to add income to the gym and they'll pay you out of that new income.

The second way is that many trainers work a second (or more) job while they're trying to get their legs at the gym. The financial strain in the beginning is pretty rough. When I started my first training job I was living at home, coming into the gym for floor hours until about 2pm, and then coaching cheerleading at night. Without needing to make rent, I had the luxury of being able to do this. Trainers who are responsible for rent often have a bunch of different jobs—they have a few clients in one gym, they teach two boot camps in another, they have a couple online clients, and they have their family friend who they train at her house every once in a while. Maybe they do some front desk hours at the gym as well. It's not a great setup. (By the way, working front desk hours is a great idea for brand new trainers. You meet every member who comes in the gym and can build natural rapport.)

There are a couple other scheduling bumps to bear in mind. The floor shifts that you want will not be available when you start. The more senior trainers will have them. The floor shifts that will be available will be either opening, closing, or weekend shifts. I can almost guarantee it. So your ass is gonna be in the gym at 5am, at 10pm, at 7am on the weekends, or possibly all three. At the beginning, I was willing to take the Friday closing shift (6pm to 9pm) and then the Saturday opening shift (6:45am to 10am) every week. It totally blows to be at the gym, close it, go to sleep, and then immediately go open it again. You feel like you've been working for two straight days and lost your entire weekend. And when you're just on floor hours, you don't really feel like you're serving a great purpose. All you know is that you're missing brunch with the girls again in order to stand around an empty gym.

But keep the faith. You are, in fact, serving a great purpose to your future self.

Because the way you get clients is by having your face in the gym all the time. Having normal conversations, doing your workouts, helping other people set their benches, showing that you generally give a shit about doing a good job at work. We'll talk about this more in future chapters, but this kind of stuff is what truly lays the foundation for your future career. People don't train with strangers. They train with people they know and trust.

You probably have a reasonable question by now. How can you be in the gym all the time if you need to work three other jobs to pay your rent? Why can't you just work from 6a to 12p every day and only take morning clients as they come along?

The short answer is: you can absolutely do this and you'll also be waiting a loooong time for those morning clients. If you're only looking to be a part-time trainer and see a few people a week, this schedule will work fine. If you're looking for full-time, it won't work fine (but everyone tries it anyway). Your master plan is to have someone at every hour from 6am to 12pm: six clients a day, five days a week, and boom! You've got 30 hours a week right there, plus you can keep the rest of your day and weekends to yourself. At our gym in 2024, this would net you an $80k annual salary. A dream!

This sounds great but fails in three ways. First, you need, like, twenty-five ideal clients for this to work. Picking up that many regular clients as a newbie can take years. Second, you can't just pick up any client. You will only be able to pick up someone who can fill in your 7am gap on Mondays and Thursdays. You'll be forced to turn down perfectly good clients in order to wait for someone who can fit your schedule perfectly. Third, people take vacations. Their kids get sick, they need to stay home for a maintenance call. You'll never have the same six sessions a day, week after week. You'd need to have clients on a waitlist who could fill last-minute gaps. There aren't many of those either.

Setting up a dream training schedule for yourself seems feasible with enough time. But, as I said before, it's not about you and your dream schedule. It's about them and their dream schedule. And it's simply not going to work any other way. I didn't believe this either. I used to leave the gym at 2pm so I could get home for my cheerleading classes at night. My boss had warned me about this, just like I'm warning you, but I ignored him, just like you're going to ignore me. He told me that leaving mid-day was going to shut off a lot of client possibilities for me. Anyone who wanted to train in the afternoons or evenings couldn't be my client.

He was right. I didn't start picking up a lot of clients until I quit my cheerleading job and stayed in the gym all day long. But once I did that? I had a full calendar within six months and started earning cash money, yo.

And, ironically, once you have a full calendar of clients is the moment when you gain one of the best parts of the job: complete schedule flexibility.

How can a trainer go from Schedule Captivity to Schedule Freedom by adding more and more people? Because your relationship with your clients will evolve to be more flexible over time. In the beginning, you give them exactly what they want for times, manage their schedule with white gloves, and gain their trust by doing great work. It's all about their time. But once people realize that you're great, they will open up their time and schedule to you. For example, they might prefer mornings generally, but because they love you and your work, they'll figure out a way to show up in the afternoon when you need them to. If you see them on Saturdays, they'll switch to Sundays when you have a gymnastics meet. As all your clients reach this point, you'll reach the holy grail of training: where you can choose the clients you want, pass along the clients who don't seem like a good fit, and scheduling becomes collaborative. Once you have loyal clients, you're not just booking the sessions they want anymore. You'll be able to take your own life and your own scheduling needs at least partially into consideration.

In this way, I can now take mornings off to write if I like, cancel my Friday night to go see *Six* on Broadway, or book a vacation, without being worried that my clients will be annoyed, or worse, leave. But there's an important caveat: my clients also know that when I'm back, I'm going to pick them right back up again, in their preferred training time slots. When I'm back, it's all about them again. We'll talk more about this in the Building Trust chapter.

Once you have a full roster of clients who trust you, you can let your schedule be anything you want. Don't want to work Fridays? Don't! You can easily fit full-time work into Mon-Thurs, and maybe a couple people on Saturday morning. Don't want to work evenings? You can easily arrange that. I hate late sessions—5pm, 6pm, especially 7pm—so as soon as I could, I stopped taking them. I lost a few of those evening clients who couldn't or wouldn't see me another time, but that's okay. When you have a strong base of clients, you can afford to lose a couple sessions a week in the name of sanity. (This is especially easy if the person you're training is an asshole. I let go of one man I saw at 6pm on Fridays, and still tell the story of when he miscounted his own sets during our workout. I pushed back, and then he said to me, "Uh...I am a math professor at Harvard University. I think I know how to count to three." I said, "Well, I also went to kindergarten, and it was two." I wasn't sad to lose him.)

If this all of this scheduling sorcery sounds workable to you, awesome! You're well on your way to becoming a great personal trainer. Let's talk about a few other pros and cons that you might not realize come along with this work.

To me, and to most trainers, the biggest pro of the job is that you are helping make people's lives better, and that's not hyperbole.

With good work, you'll help them move more easily, with less pain, in greater quantities than they used to. Their health and capacity will improve. And the more they love working with you, the more they'll start doing it on their own, which is my personal ambition for every client. They come to see me, learn a shit-ton about their bodies and their health, and then take that information and carry it with them forever, whether they keep training with me or not. It's beautiful to watch. Do not—DO NOT—do that bullshit where you purposely build their dependence on your work, so that your clients feel like they can't lift a finger without you. That's gross.

Here are some other pros of the job, and there are a lot of them:

- **Building incredible friendships with your clients and other gym members.** Many of my closest friends are people who started as clients (and most of them are still clients today). As a trainer, you spend more one-on-one time with people than they do with almost anyone else in their lives. It's natural that you become fast friends, and, frankly, it's almost essential. You don't have to hang out with everyone you train, but the personality match needs to be there. More on this in the chapter on nurturing client relationships.

• **Developing a network.** Different from friendships, this is just the sheer number of people who will be willing to help you down the road. This is part of the reward that comes from spending your beginning years in servitude to others. When you give so much of yourself away, people will want to pay you back when the time comes. My business partners and I have been lucky enough to use our own networks in a number of ways to get our gym, Amplify Fitness, off the ground. And we aren't the first trainers to say that.

• **Personal training fosters entrepreneurship.** A ton of career trainers go on to open small gyms, start online businesses, franchise big chains, or become independent of a gym and work privately. All of this comes from building great relationships with your clients and putting in the effort to give them what they want. If you've always tried to help them, they'll be thrilled to help you too.

• **Access to excellent, cheap education.** Most personal training conferences aren't very expensive and many gyms will help offset the costs of attending. The big conferences in the industry are largely hosted by blowhards (you can read more of my venom on this in the Thoughts On The Industry chapter), but there are tons of small conferences that are fantastic. You can also read research online for free, check out the textbooks that are inevitably sitting in every staff office, get continuing education credits (CEU's, necessary to maintain an active PT certification), etc. Not to mention, anywhere you work will have one of the best educational opportunities you could ask for: your coworkers. Learning from other trainers is a gold mine, and you should pounce on every opportunity to talk with them. The world of fitness is infinite, and great knowledge is not restricted to experienced trainers. Everyone has a different life experience that brought them to personal training. I didn't have a day of training experience in my life but there I was, a new trainer, teaching my coworkers how to do handstands. Always remember that every human on the planet knows things that you don't know.

• **Every hour of your work is different.** If you have ADHD, this is a dream job! Every day of work will be different than every previous day. The variety is wonderful for those of us who get depressed when everything is monotone. Even doing 1500 sessions a year, I'm rarely bored. People's bodies are always doing new and interesting things, and the people themselves always have new and interesting things to tell you about.

• **You'll become a master of pivoting.** There are always surprises in training. Like the people who come in and say, "Hey, I didn't have a chance to let you know, but I broke six bones in my foot last week and have to stay off of it today." Like, what? So much for our agility plan today and our agility program for the next twelve weeks. Or the people who come in and say, "My period is trying to murder me. Can we please lie on the ground for sixty minutes?" You'll get extremely good at thinking on your feet and instantly pivoting a session. This also helps me in real life all the time. When plans change or get totally fucked up somewhere, I am always the coolest one in the group. It doesn't faze me in the least. I can go an entirely new direction on a dime, and I probably also have four other ideas we can implement immediately. Keeping things moving no matter what is going on is a trainer speciality, and probably the most important skill a trainer can develop.

- **You'll never need to work at a desk.** Fuck working at a desk. It would literally destroy me. This profession is a guarantee that that will never happen to you.

- **Great job security.** This is true about service jobs in general. People will always want services in their lives and the more they hear about you, the more they'll want to work with you. (Think of how you can't wait to go to a restaurant that everyone keeps talking about.) I've kept a running wait list for at least ten years now (not with the same people on it, omg), and hope to be lucky enough to continue that for a long time.

- **People give you things.** I've never expected tips from anyone, but they've always come in, especially during the holidays. Over the years, clients and gym members have been extremely kind to me, offering me gifts like time in their vacation homes, airplane upgrades, electronic and tech gadgets, even loaning me cars when my car has broken down. I've gone to fancy dinners, met celebrities, and attended premier sporting events and concerts. Let's be clear: this is NOT why you should become a personal trainer. I never expected a single one of these things (who would??), and I still don't expect them now. But the fact is, again, that when you do your best to provide someone with something that enriches their lives, they will often want to thank you. It is deeply humbling.

- **Salary commissions are excellent.** For as much as your salary sucks in the beginning, it gets better and better as you go. First of all, most gyms have a sliding scale, where you get paid more per session when you do more sessions. In other words, if you do 1-10 sessions in the pay period, you might earn $28 per session. But if you do 65+ sessions in the pay period, you would earn $52 per session. Huge difference. Most gyms also have sales bonuses each month to encourage client retention, and also session bonuses per pay period. Our old gym paid $100 extra per pay period if you did more than 60 sessions in those two weeks. As long as you're never trying to con your clients into doing extra sessions just so you can get your bonus, this system works great. I always felt motivated to add in sessions to my workload, without feeling like I was using my clients for cash. More on this in the cons below, and also in the client retention chapters.

One last pro of the job? You work in a gym. That means two things for your own exercise. Number one, it's free, which is a big deal for someone like you who uses a gym frequently. Fitness is expensive. Number two, it's as convenient as exercise will ever be. You'll already be there, and you'll be able to take advantage of ten free minutes as easily as you can take advantage of two free hours.

So that's a lot of pros for this job. But what are the biggest cons of being a personal trainer?

For me, one of the big negatives of my job is providing an excellent service to a difficult person, especially if they are insulting or demeaning. When you're just starting out, you're going to need to say yes to every single session if you want to make money, and sometimes that means saying yes to people you REALLY don't like working with. As you get a bigger client base, you'll feel financially comfortable enough to divorce the clients who are rude to you and just keep the great ones. But in the beginning, unfortunately, you're gonna get some duds. Like the Author/Filmmaker, with her BMW keys and her thrown coats and her demands for wakeup calls.

Nearly all of the other cons have to do with money, unfortunately. Here they are:

- **The salary in the beginning.** Yes, you can make a lot of money as a trainer. But in the beginning your salary is only your floor hours, and however many sessions you did during that pay period. When you have just one or two clients, it's pretty grim. In our gym, I always feel guilty that I can't pay our trainers more at the outset. Unfortunately, there isn't really a better way of doing it. No gym has the extra cash to pay all their trainers a large salary at the start, plus there isn't much work to pay them for. They only have work once they have clients.

- **No benefits at the start.** This goes along with the salary issues. I can't speak for every gym here, but our old gym would only give trainers benefits once they started making full-time hours. I didn't have benefits for years. Then, after you get benefits, they audit you every three months. If you don't average thirty-five training hours a week? Your benefits are cut immediately until the next audit. That includes if you averaged 34.999999999 hours (and I saw this happen to a few coworkers). The savviest among us were always obsessively checking our hours, adding and moving sessions around in order to be sure we'd stay above water. But this has its own issues:

- **You can never take much time off.** If I took a day off from work, I knew I'd need to make up those eight to ten hours somewhere else. If I were taking a Friday off, I would try my hardest to rearrange all of my Friday clients into other days. What this means is that a day off is never actually a day off. You're just cramming that day's work into other days instead.

You don't want to cram? Then you better be watching those benefits hours like a hawk. Going away for more than a week? I don't think I did that in the entire twelve years that I worked at my old gym. It would have meant benefits suicide. You can make up a few days of vacation with some schedule finesse. It's nearly impossible to make up sixty to eighty hours of vacation in a three-month audit period.

• **Your earnings will always be unpredictable, no matter how successful you are.** When you're an hourly employee who creates their own hours, you never know how big your next check will be. This is almost always what tanked the career hopes of trainers who were also parents. It's hard to provide for kids when you don't know how much you're earning this month. Typically, my biggest months of the year were January, March, and October. Few holidays, thirty-one days, unpopular travel times. Easy to maintain forty to forty-five sessions a week. My worst months were July, August, and December, when everyone is away for long periods of time. In these three months I might only make twenty to thirty sessions a week, and that's with a full client list. Before I had a full client list, I had some Augusts where I dropped to five sessions a week. You will have to learn to prepare for leaner checks by being smart about your bigger checks.

• **Working forty hours a week in a service job means forty hours of work.** You might be used to a desk job, where you get lunch breaks, work from home, chatting time around the coffee maker, summer Fridays, and plenty of opportunities to sit on your phone texting friends, playing Wordle, heckling the other managers in your fantasy leagues, online shopping, etc. Working full-time in personal training means forty full hours of work, not just forty hours of being in the building. (You're usually in the building for much longer than that, because sessions don't always line up for the entire day.)

The other full-time trainers and I rarely ate, generally sneaking a few bites at the top of the hour just after one client finished and the next was tying their sneakers. I would usually give a client instructions to start their warm-up, run to pee (or omg if I had to poop it was so stressful), and then try to be back within 90 seconds, before they felt like their money was being wasted. It is MUCH more work time than many professions. I might go eight hours without checking my phone, and then have a bunch of people annoyed with me for being hard to reach or unresponsive. If you're coming from another career, you might be shocked by how much time forty hours of work truly is.

• **You always need to be on.** You're having a bad day? Too bad. You need to be warm, friendly, inviting, carefree, focused on giving an excellent session for every client, every day. You don't talk about your problems, you ask about their problems. You don't complain about your sore knee, you ask about their sore knees. Much like a therapist, you're there to listen to your client and let them have their hour for themselves. They're not booking time with you to talk about you. Sure, many clients will ask you questions, because they're normal humans having normal conversations. But I will always try to bring the conversation back to them before too long.

Part of the joy of personal training on the client side is that they feel like it's a special hour that they're taking for themselves, where nothing else in their life can touch them. If you've ever gone to get a massage or a facial and had a provider who talked the whole time about themselves, then you can understand exactly why you shouldn't be doing that. It's incredibly distracting. And as much as Gen Z is gonna hate this, you can't cancel sessions because you're having a bad day either. For traumatic stuff? Of course cancel. But you fought with your girlfriend, you had a flat tire late at night, you have terrible period pain, you sprained your ankle, you got upsetting news, you have a hangover, it doesn't matter. You need to show up anyway, and you need to be "on". Consistency is the most important quality to have in any service field. People need to know that you will always be there. If you're not, they will leave. (Or you will get fired. Fast.)

• **People will always ask you when you're going to get a real job.** This one is so fucking infuriating. Job snobbery is real, and people think that working in a gym isn't a real job. They think it's something that stupid, aimless people do. Even when I had been a full-time trainer for many years, earning plenty of money, I still had people asking me when I was going to stop messing around and get a real job. Even a few of my own clients would do this in a more subtle way. Hey, just for the record? If you do work and get paid for it, you have a real job.

The summary of life as a personal trainer is that in the beginning, your schedule will be fucked and you will not make any money or have any benefits. If you can tough that out, use the extra time for education, and get a bunch of clients, your schedule will become all yours. You'll eventually get benefits, and you will make plenty of money for as long as you're willing to keep nurturing your client relationships. There's no upper limit on sessions either. I don't recommend this, but if you want to work eighty sessions a week, no one is stopping you. You can literally make as much money as you want.

If I haven't scared you away, then let's dive in. The rest of this book talks about everything else: choosing a certification and passing your exam, meeting and assessing new clients, maintaining excellent client relationships (AKA keeping a pristine reputation), creating and updating exercise programs, handling the thorny money and business questions that arise, generating sales, my thoughts on the industry at large (grab your popcorn for this one), and individual chapter summary Do's and Don'ts, for everyone who suffers from TL;DR syndrome. If there's a chapter that you already feel experienced in, feel free to skip to the summary TL;DR at the end.

Now, let's get you certified.

TL; DR:

1) Be prepared to donate a lot of your time and schedule to the gym in the beginning of your career. You're gonna feel like you're just sitting around a lot, because you are. It will suck. That's just how it goes.

2) It is critical that you really, really love to watch people move around. If you find everything about movement interesting, a career in general fitness will be a superb match for you. If you're only interested in certain types of movement, head for a gym that matches your vibe. If you're only really into it when people are 1RMing a back squat, you will do much better in a powerlifting gym than a big box cheapo gym. If you're mostly into sadistic death cardio, head to Crossfit or similar. If you're only interested in teaching rehab, consider physical therapy, occupational therapy, or athletic training instead. Seeking out a gym environment that you love will help you deal with all the initial sitting around, because it'll still be fun to be there watching.

3) The clients always come first. Their schedule, their workouts, their goals, and their bad moods. You need to be invested in every session as much as possible, no matter how grumpy or distracted you are by other things. They can be in a bad mood the whole time; you can't.

Chapter Three: Getting Certified

So, you've decided you can deal with earning shit money for a while and you're ready to start training. Sweet! LFG.

The first question: what kind of education do you need to get your foot in the door?

The "ideal" trainer, according to generic employers, has a bachelor's degree in exercise science/physiology/kinesiology/another related field, and a national PT certification. If you're hoping to work in collegiate or professional athletics, you're going to need a degree (possibly an advanced one) and a CSCS (certified strength and conditioning specialist—the most-valued PT certification). Those are non-negotiable, unless you're a nepobaby or grandfathered in by being famous in your sport. But just to be clear: you absolutely do not need to have an exercise degree, or any college degree, to be a great personal trainer. (My own degree is in French Language and Literature, donc vous pouvez voir pourquoi je m'en fiche.)

If you don't have a degree in a related field, then you'll need a personal training certification to get a job. And even if you do have a degree, you'll still get a certification on top of that, because employers like to see them. So the certification is your first step. You'll want one that's accredited by the NCCA (National Commission for Certifying Agencies), and fortunately, there are plenty. The NCCA doesn't actually offer the certification; they simply recognize the validity of several different companies and their training certs.

There are a trillion companies who promise online personal training certifications in a weekend, no test required, stamped in crayon, just give them $500 and they'll put your name on a fancy napkin. Don't do this. Get off the internet. Homer Simpson yourself backwards into the bushes, and go get a real cert from an accredited body.

The most common and most well-respected certifications are:

- ACE (American Council of Exercise)

- NASM (National Academy of Sports Medicine)

- NSCA (National Strength and Conditioning Association)

- ACSM (American College of Sports Medicine)

- ISSA (International Sports Sciences Association)

- NFPT (National Federation of Personal Trainers)

The first four are the biggest ones. The last two are slightly lesser-known but are still accredited and will easily land you a job anywhere. As with anything, all of the certs have their pros and cons. The following are my crude descriptions, but generally accurate. ACE is thought of as the easiest to pass because it keeps the info relatively basic; I always find myself wanting more detail from them. NSCA is thought of as the most difficult to pass, because it has the most scientific strength and conditioning focus, but is not as strong in teaching about groups that aren't young men. NASM is sort of a little-piece-of-everything, lot-of-piece-of-nothing type of cert, and ACSM is strong in their special populations coaching (pre/post-natal, seniors, etc) but weaker in their strength and conditioning coaching. ISSA is strong in S&C but also super expensive. NFPT costs the least, but is pretty entry-level overall.

When I was starting out, I asked everyone I met what the hardest certification to get was, because that's the one I wanted to get. (This is just the type of annoying person that I am.) Everyone unequivocally agreed that NSCA was it. So I got their CPT and, eventually, their

CSCS as well. I passed both on the first try, although I was miffed that I did not get a perfect score on either (again, because I'm an annoying person).

If you're not annoying, all of these certs will be just fine. I don't know of any gyms who prefer ACSM's CPT over NASM's CPT, for example, or any other preference. The big certification companies are big business—I get tired of their loud website graphics and endless sales pitches for the smaller, more specialized certs that they offer—but all of them will teach you plenty of information to get your career started. I spent 3-6 months studying for each one, and didn't find either certification to be particularly difficult to pass.

You can usually buy the certifying exam by itself for three to five hundred bucks, with no obligation to buy their textbooks, practice exams, or other study materials. If you pass, you're good to go. But I don't recommend this route for a couple reasons. The first reason is that although most people with a general understanding of fitness should be able to pass these exams, a trainer must be better than general. So even if you can pass the exam right off the bat, you still have to learn more. Take your time, study well, and learn some shit you didn't know. Be better than general.

The second reason to use extra study materials is that these exams aren't always based on the exact same fitness research and knowledge. They are based on what the governing body itself teaches. In other words, the NSCA exam is based on the NSCA textbook. The ACE exam is based on the ACE textbook. I was an experienced trainer when I decided to get my CSCS, and I failed multiple practice exams during my study time. I couldn't figure out why until I got the CSCS-specific textbook. Many of the test questions came directly from it and were slightly different from what I had been taught in other places. As soon as I read it, I passed my next practice exam easily. The certifying bodies don't write tests based on the most-accepted practice. They ask questions about what *they specifically teach in their book*. There's obviously plenty of overlap, but not 100%. So don't rely on your general knowledge, and don't use one text to study for another test.

I would allocate about a thousand dollars and several months to get your personal training certification. The exam, the books, and the practice exams are all worth buying. I own most of the certifying body textbooks and I read them regularly. They're excellent primers on the many fields that make up the world of exercise—biomechanics, physiology, anatomy, nutrition—while being easier to read than any given textbook in any of those fields. They also cover ideas like client assessment, programming, and behavioral coaching, if that helps you. I personally discovered that studying human behavior is much, much easier when you are studying an actual human in front of you, not the hypothetical case studies in a book, but always do what works for you.

(Related: I have learned multiple styles of client-assessment techniques from certifications, the internet, my bosses, and conferences. In the end, the very best client-assessment technique is laughably simple: have a conversation with the person. I write about this in detail in the first Client Assessment chapter.)

Here's the biggest downfall of all of the certifications: you will become a personal trainer and realize you still don't really know anything about personal training. There is an enormous gap between answering exam questions successfully and having a full-sized human relying on you to keep them safe, healthy, and progressing in the gym.

This isn't specific to personal training; No doctor gets their MD and feels confident diving into residency. No physical therapist finishes a DPT and feels prepared to provide competent care. And that's after three to four years of rigorous education. (Rigorous might be a gentle way of describing the near-death experience of med school but here we are.) Personal trainers, although working equally closely with people who need help, don't have the same educational background and degree requirements. We go into the field extremely green. This is one reason why other health fields often deride personal trainers as being dangerous garbage frauds. I go into this weird dynamic in great detail in the chapter on collaborative care.

(Incidentally, Dangerous Garbage Frauds is gonna be the name of my upcoming derivative folk album.)

If you don't have an Exercise Science degree, then you will have, at best, a couple months of self-guided education in order to get your CPT. It's not enough. You will feel like you have absolutely no idea what to do with a new client, and you would be right. Don't worry! That's why I wrote this book. I wanted to add some field knowledge that isn't taught in textbooks. I will help you figure out assessments, safe starting workout plans, and develop a business acumen that won't fail you. But also: you need to learn more on your own. Constantly. Have I mentioned that?

For now, just worry about passing your exam and deciding on your specialties. Do some research on the major certifying bodies and choose the one that sounds best for you.

Now, let's go over the extra certifications. There are a ton just within the four primary certifying bodies alone. Group Exercise, Senior Fitness, Childhood Fitness, Pre/Post Natal Fitness, Health Coach, Medical Exercise Specialist, Tactical Strength, Functional Strength, Corrective Exercise, Wellness Coach, Women's Fitness, Nutrition Counselor, etc etc etc.

And outside of the big companies, there are a zillion other companies who offer certs as well. Functional Movement Specialist, Functional

Range Conditioning, Z-Health, Crossfit, Strong First, RKC, USAW, and on and on forever and ever and ever.

So, do you need them?

Short answer, no. You don't **need** any of these.

You can definitely get your CPT, get a job, get field experience, and just keep renewing that cert every two years until you stop training. Some gyms will increase your pay if you get more certifications, but not all. Following this path is perfectly fine for people who intend to work in general fitness. The general fitness population is *huge*. With a CPT and time, you'll have no issues being an effective coach for them.

If you want to target a certain population, or specialize in something like Olympic weightlifting, kettlebells, mobility, etc, it'll be well-worth your time to get a specialty cert. Mostly because clients looking for a kettlebell coach are going to wonder if you've really put in the time to understand kettlebells on an advanced level, or if you're just another CPT who's passing along kettlebell tips from Instagram. An RKC or SFG will reassure people that you've spent time, money, and effort on bells.

I would get specialty certs from the independent companies, not the giants.

Here's the truth: most specialty certifications from the big four fitness companies add very little to your resumé. They offer them because they want their CPT's to return to get more certifications (which then need to be re-certified every couple years). Like King George, they're counting on your brand loyalty forever and ever and ever. It's not that their certs are useless and I'm not trying to shit on them. But in my opinion, if you want to specialize in something, then you want a cert from a specialty. You want a mobility cert from people who only sell mobility certs. You want to learn kettlebell work from someone who's obsessed with kettlebells. Remember, the big four companies are (for good reason) essentially jacks-of-all-trades when it comes to fitness. They want to teach you a bit of everything so you can be as best prepared for the general fitness field as you can be. But a jack-of-all-trades is a master of none. If you want to be a master, then go to a master.

No matter how you get it, you will need continuing education, and some of it will need to be done by yourself. This comes through reading, studying, and learning extra on your own, outside of all of the certifications. Everyone who sells a cert—big four and specialty—is convinced that their way is the only way. They want to teach you one thing: their thing. They'll tell you that everything else is less important. This is unavoidable in fitness, and it's also dead wrong. Human bodies come in a huge array, and you will be caring for many of them. One cert or specialty isn't gonna cover the variety of people you'll see in your career. Kettlebells will be brilliant for one client and intolerable for another. A third will refuse to use them and a fourth will try but never understand the movements well enough for them to be effective. You'll always need backup ideas and techniques for when what you're doing isn't working.

I have collected a bunch of certs over the years, some that I think are valuable and some that I do not. My certs absolutely do not reflect my capabilities as a trainer, and yours won't either. For example, I am a senior fitness expert without a senior fitness certification. It's one of my strongest training skills, learned entirely in the field. There is no certification on the planet that could have adequately prepared me for the challenges and joys of training the (hundred or so) seventy, eighty, and ninety-year-olds that I've worked with in my career. That experience is now worth much more on my resumé than any senior fitness cert would be.

No matter the topic, no certification is more valuable than long hours spent carefully watching people move around. I would rather watch the human bodies in front of me, read current papers, listen to what today's experts are lecturing on, study my own movement, and attend great conferences, than spend endless money getting more and more certifications. Just know that certs are one way of educating and specializing yourself, not the only way.

Speaking of specialties. No matter how you do it, you'll want to figure out what you're good at and then start homing in on that. Don't be fooled into thinking that you'll be the best trainer for every human being on Earth. We all think that in the beginning, and we're all wrong. Trainer ego. Amateur hour.

Specializing will help you find the right clients for you. Almost no one who is looking for a trainer will be able to identify what kind of trainer she wants or needs. Most people think that exercise is basic, uncomplicated, and the same for everybody, so they won't know the difference between trainers. I remember one client being astonished that I was attending a conference that was three days long. He said, "There's enough exercise in the world to spend three straight days talking about it?" Sir, I would attend a three-day conference exclusively about hip extension, are you kidding me? Another client couldn't understand how I was once writing an article about pistol squats. "How is there enough information about pistol squats to write a whole article? Don't you just go down and go up?" Yes, in the same way that an article about cars wouldn't need to say anything besides "Turn it on and drive."

Exercise, like everything in the human body, is anything but basic and uncomplicated. I know you know this, because people who want to be trainers have already been influenced by one type of exercise and coaching that spoke to them. That specificity is what you're now looking to bring to someone else. But since the average gym-goer doesn't know about specificity in exercise, they won't know how to look for you. You need to be on the lookout for them. Keep an eye out for people who are practicing the thing that you teach, and then bring them on board with you. Again, it's not going to be every single client in the gym. You're not right for everyone. If you wouldn't choose a surgeon who cheerfully says, "Oh, I just cut into everything!", then don't be a trainer who says, "Oh, I can train you for anything!"

Narrowing down your training focus to the few things that you coach the best, like the best, and understand the best is going to be one of your biggest assets. Trust me, this is way better than pretending like you can coach any athlete under the sun. First of all, the sheer confidence to think you could. Second of all, a person who sells to everyone sells to no one. You need to have your specific thing that you're great at, and then sell that to the people who want to buy it.

How do you know what you're great at? Start by looking at your past.

All trainers have a type of training modality, a sport, a joint or body area, a core belief, memorable moments, and individual values that guide their own view of exercise. It's what makes personal training such a cool field. Trainers will inevitably draw on their lived experiences as an integral part of what they teach to clients, and they should! Teach what you know.

My lived experience is in gymnastics, cheerleading, ninja warrior, and track. My specialities are advanced bodyweight conditioning, basic weight training, gymnastics-based skills like handstands, pullups, swinging, mobility, flexibility, and balance. I also really love spines, shoulders, and hips—my favorite joints. I know more about them than any other joints, so I naturally gravitate towards people who have lingering problems in those areas. I also deeply believe that there is a type of movement out there for every human on the planet. This belief helps me connect with beginners who don't know what kind of exercise might appeal to them. This combination of skills and values is what I bring to my clients who are looking for exactly what I know and what I can teach.

I would never accept a client who wanted to bodybuild, or who wanted long-distance running programs from me, or who wanted to compete in high-level powerlifting, or who wanted to become a proficient Olympic lifter. I can teach the basics of all of those modalities, but I'm not an expert in any of them. If I took a client for one of those modalities under the hubris that my basic knowledge was good enough, I'm doing everyone a disservice. Instead, I'm going to set them up with one of our trainers who is an expert in those modalities. And if one of those trainers gets approached by someone with stiff hips who wants to join an adult dodgeball team, they're gonna send them straight to me.

Not only does this get the best fit between client and trainer, but also eliminates the distrust that some gyms create between trainers. You're never in competition with each other if everyone is treated as a unique contributor to the team. I've heard some horror stories about client poaching (trying to steal another trainer's clients when the trainer goes on vacation or calls out sick) and y'all, do NOT go work in a gym that encourages that trash. It's despicable for everyone: trainers won't trust their coworkers and clients get treated like nothing more than a wallet. It also reinforces the concept that all trainers are the same, therefore one is entirely expendable and replaceable by another.

Side note while we're here: I don't trust gyms whose sole focus is on selling as much personal training as possible. You can pick them out because they bill all their trainers as being WICKED AMAZING AT EVERYTHING. It's a con. Trust in gyms who sit down with their clients, ask them what they're looking for, and take the time to set them up with a good training match. The same goes for physical therapy places, by the way. All physical therapists get training on all joints, but providers should have specialties and interests. Give me an ankle expert when my ankle is broken. Give me a shoulder expert when my shoulder is broken. I won't even go to a PT clinic if the receptionist says, "Oh, all of our therapists can treat anything." Boo, hiss, throw tomatoes. Just like how you want to learn kettlebells from people who are obsessed with kettlebells, you want to get your shoulder cared for by someone who is obsessed with shoulders. This should be basic but it's not, because companies don't like turning away business.

At our gym, and all the gyms I've been lucky enough to work at, we encourage specialities. Yes, it takes longer to build a full client base, because clients are paired with the trainers we think fit them best, not just the first available. But the tradeoff is happy clients being trained by happy trainers. Everyone sticks around longer, which is good for the client, good for the trainer, and good for the gym. In the long run, it's a no-brainer.

So, how should you choose your specialties? Several of them could be chosen for you based on your lived experience. Did you do gymnastics? Then bodyweight conditioning is familiar. Track? You've got a running or jumping specialty. Football? Agility, power. Didn't do any sports growing up and got into fitness later? You're gonna be excellent at training beginners because you know where they're coming from. Lost or gained body mass? You know what it takes. I do so many pull-ups that training women to do pull-ups became an extremely easy specialty for me.

Outside of lived experience, you will find that some groups of people simply appeal to you the most. I get so much joy out of working with ninety-year-olds. No one else is as wise and funny as they are, plus they're so badass and few people recognize that. I also love Try-Hards. A client might be so beginner that we spend sixty minutes trying to sit to a block and stand up one time, but if they are trying as hard as they can, I'm riveted. Some trainers don't want beginners. They want elite athletes, because they thrive on those tiny adjustments that can shave a tenth of a second off of a sprint. Other trainers love watching people move big ass weights. Still others are interested in pain, and they become the desperately-needed bridge in healthcare between physical therapy and return to sport.

Wherever you land, you'll have people looking for your skills. So don't worry that your niche is gonna be too small, or that you're going to miss out on clients. The world is huge, and a lot of people need help with their fitness. Yes, it'll take you a little longer to find your people. But when you find them, they're going to stick with you for a long, long time. Some of my clients have trained with me for fifteen years.

One other note about certifications, both to future trainers and employers who might be reading this. Field experience is difficult to quantify and difficult to put on a resumé. It is a mistake to assume someone is a better trainer because they have more certifications than someone else. What a trainer can do with a client is what's most important: can they motivate them appropriately, listen to them carefully, train them safely, and guide them confidently. Certifications are only letters on a page until they are put into good practice.

And speaking of letters on a page, if you've seen me lecture anywhere, you might have seen my own PowerPoint title page, which reads:

Mia Lazarewicz

co-founder, Amplify Fitness Boston

NSCA-CPT, CSCS, SFB, Z-Health, CFB

Those are my CPT, my CSCS, my SFB (StrongFirst Bodyweight certification), and my Z-Health mobility certifications (I've done a few with them). And the CFB? It stands for Certified Fucking Badass. At first, I had started adding this to my resumé as a commentary on how stupid it was to assume that a person is smart just because they have a bunch of letters after their name. But as time went on, I realized it was probably my most important designation of the bunch. A certification I awarded to myself long ago, which will renew indefinitely at the low cost of refusing to be anything else.

Feel free to steal this certification for yourself, no textbooks, practice exams, or fees needed. And don't stress too much about your other certs. Get your CPT and get going. You can add everything else on the way.

TL; DR:

1) The big four certifications are more or less the same for CPTs. I have never met a gym owner who demanded that all their trainers have a certain certification. The only exception to this is the CSCS, which is a non-negotiable for most high-level coaching positions.

2) Bachelor's degree in a related field is nice but not necessary. Accessory certifications are nice but not necessary.

3) Remember that certifications are only a part of what makes you a great, well-educated trainer. Your time in the field, ability to read and apply current research, attendance at interesting conferences, self-exercise practice, personal lived experience, and professionalism will all matter more than your certifications ever can.

Chapter Four: How To Meet Clients

One of the most perplexing parts of being a new trainer is: Where the fuck are you gonna get clients from?

No one knows you. Why would anyone train with you, especially when it's so expensive? How do they know if you're any good? Frankly, how will they even know you exist?

I will never forget my first client. (Whitney, sending you love! You changed everything for me.) We met when she signed up for membership and was automatically assigned to me for her complimentary appointments. We chatted for our first session, we did a workout for our second session, and when that workout was done, I said, "Have you given any thought to personal training?" At this point I had probably met with eight or ten prospectives and none of them had any interest in training with me, so I had zero expectations. But she said, "You know, I think I'm going to try the pack of eight sessions."

I was so surprised I literally said, "Wait, seriously????" which, by the way, is not the most professional response. There are better answers. But I was so excited! Someone wanted to work out with me! We trained for a few years until she left for medical school and I will always be grateful that she took a chance on me. Getting your first client gives you a ton of confidence. You learned enough about them, gave them a good workout, and convinced them that your service is valuable. That's awesome. And if you can convince someone to buy PT when you're a baby trainer, just think how much easier it will be when you have more experience.

Whitney was assigned to me by our sales staff, which is a common way to meet prospective clients. For gyms that offer complimentary training sessions, as soon as a new member signs up, they are put in contact with a trainer. Some gyms do this cyclically—the next member goes to Sean, and then the one after that goes to Mia, and the one after that goes to Eric. This ensures that all trainers get approximately the same number of prospectives. Some gyms, like ours, try to evaluate the best fit and get people set up with the trainer who best matches their needs. Other gyms have no pipeline at all, and their trainers are expected to get new clients by a wing and a prayer. Use caution when accepting a position at this type of gym.

But, even if there is a feed from sales, if you sit around waiting for the gym to send you clients, it's gonna take you all of eternity to fill your client list. For one thing, lots of new members will never book their free sessions. Unfortunately, they don't see the value in them. They think it's just a two-hour, multiple-day, money-making scheme for the gym. *Hi there! Do you have some time to hear about this timeshare in Florida?* It's not that way (or rather, shouldn't be), but some people will never believe that.

For another thing, some new members will book one session, not show up (because it's free and they don't care), waste your time, book it for another week, show up, take two months to book the second session, and then tell you they don't want training they just want you to create a six-month, individualized, program for them to work out five days a week on their own and could you just email it to them when you get a chance?

(Baby trainers, when this happens to you—and it will happen all the time—practice saying, "I'd be happy to do that. It will take me four to five hours to develop that for you. Are you interested in a six-pack of sessions to cover the cost? We can use the sixth session to go over the entire program in person.")

Fortunately, there are tons of ways to meet clients that don't involve waiting for the gym to send you people. The first one is your trainer bio.

Most gyms with steadily-employed personal trainers will have a PT bio wall. Each trainer's picture is shown along with their training interests, capabilities, and background. Do not waste your bio space! This is a huge opportunity to get people to come to you without you doing a single extra thing. Think of your bio as passive income. Once you create a great one, it will continue generating revenue for you for years. My old bio had a space for a favorite quote. Lots of other trainers wrote stuff about motivation, dedication, or drive. Mine? It said, "Who needs buns of steel? I'd rather have buns of cinnamon." A legendary Ellen Degeneres quote. I got a half-dozen long-term clients specifically because that quote made them want to meet me.

My current bio at the gym mentions that I'm an expert in bodyweight conditioning, mobility, gymnastics, and balance training. It also mentions that I used to live in France, that I've sat at Emeril's table in New Orleans, and that I've competed on American Ninja Warrior. People ask me about these last three things way more than the first four things. It's a simple way to maximize your exposure to every member at the gym. And if you say something interesting in your bio, I guarantee people will come find you to talk about it.

The bio is super helpful passively, but what's the best way to actively meet new potential clients? Teach group exercise classes, especially when you're new. I got a TON of clients over the years from my classes. Many of those people still train with me today. It was also common for class attendees to occasionally book one or two sessions because they wanted to practice something that came up in class. Never turn your nose up at one or two sessions. If you have a dozen people who want to train once a month, that's the same as two or three full-time clients. And never turn your nose up anyway. People need help, and you have the power to provide help. So provide it.

In addition to teaching your own regular classes when possible, accept every opportunity to sub a class for someone else. When you sub someone else's class, you meet a dozen new people who have never trained with you before. If they like your sub class, they'll start coming to your real classes too. They'll also be interested in your training. And tell their friends about you. Furthermore, when a class finishes, most of the attendees go straight to the locker room to debrief. You know who will be listening in on their gossip sesh? Every other person in the locker room. Word of mouth is the gold standard recommendation. I've gotten plenty of clients from secondhand locker room chatter.

Are you getting the gist here? As soon as people know what you can do, they're going to want to train with you. It might not be right now, which is fine. They will show up eventually. That's something else I learned along the way: even if you've piqued someone's interest, they rarely come straight to you. No, no. That would be too easy and too normal. What they do instead is silently watch you, follow you, and listen to you from the side. Constantly. Sometimes for years.

You will be watched by other people in the gym in every single session that you do. They will watch the exercises your client is doing and then imitate them off to the side. They will listen in on your conversations. They will laugh at the jokes you thought you made to just one person. They will imagine themselves doing the workout your client is doing and wonder if they would be able to do it. All of this will happen without you realizing it, until someone comes up to you and tells you they've been watching you for a year and finally decided they want to work with you. Often it's because they want to be sure you're worth the money. I have one fantastic client who, I learned later, evaluated me for *years* before ever saying a single word to me. For others, the wait is not because of a doubt in your abilities, but rather a fear of them. One woman told me it took her more than a year to gather the courage to come to my class because it looked so scary from the outside. But after trying once, she attended twice weekly for eight years.

Here's another excellent way to pick up new clients: talk to people. Say hello to gym members you haven't met. Ask people about their workouts, their weekend plans, their families. The next time you see them, ask them how the apple picking was, or how their son's birthday party went. This isn't to lure them into working with you, it's called being a human. Show genuine interest in people and their lives. Some of those people will remember that you're a friendly, thoughtful person and you'll be the first one they think of when they decide they're in the market for a trainer. Personal training is a long game, not a short one. People will come to you when they're ready.

There's one last great way to meet members and potential clients: doing your own workouts at work. Chances are you're an experienced athlete in some respects, or you wouldn't want this job. I didn't know this when I started, but once people find out you're a trainer, they will watch your workouts like a hawk. My box jumps and my pull-ups started a lot of conversations with people, especially women who wanted to learn those skills.

Almost any workout you do is going to trigger notice. It's like how people want to know what a nutritionist is eating, or what type of car a mechanic drives. Less-conventional workouts are an attention gold mine. Creative kettlebell work, battle ropes, agility ladders, sled pushing, handstands, treadmill hill runs, and clever station setups can all generate buzz. I didn't always let this guide my workout programming, but when the gym was packed, did I try to set up my highest box jumps right in the middle? Yes, yes I absolutely did. And you know what? One of my clients recently said to me, "Remember when we first met and you were doing those absolutely insane jumps?"

It's flattering that she was impressed, but the real point here is that my workout gave us a reason to talk in the first place.

Why do your workouts have such an impact on people? Like it or not, your body is one of the things people evaluate when they are trying to decide if you're a good trainer. I'm not talking about the size of your body, although unfortunately there are still a few small-minded douchecanoes out there who care if you're thin. Ignore them. You're not doing workouts to show new clients that you're thin. It's much more about people seeing that you are strong. Everyone wants to be strong.

You have to be strong to be a trainer. I don't really mean your muscles, even though that helps. Strength is a limitless entity, and we call on many kinds of strength in every workout. So if you're not jacked AF, that's not the point. The point is that while a trainer does need to understand what makes a physically strong body, they also need to understand what makes a mentally strong body. Resilience; empathy; getting uncomfortable; trusting yourself; testing your mental capacity; how to wallow in the mud when you're really going through it. These all matter, you'll reflect these things in your own workouts, and other people will notice. They'll notice that you're resilient in your own workouts, empathetic to your own struggles, and assume that you'll be the same way for them (which you will be).

People will like it if you're a physically strong trainer. Walking the walk and talking the talk, as it were. But no matter how physically strong you are, your giant delts can't do the pushups for your client. So when I say that people are evaluating your body, yes, some of them will only ever judge your capabilities based on what you look like. But most of them are secretly evaluating your spirit in the gym, not your talent. They want to see you grinding it out, missing lifts and going back for more, challenging yourself to eke out another pull-up. They want to see you take yourself seriously, but not pout or break shit when it goes wrong.

More than anything, they want to see you trying. Because they know, maybe subconsciously, that the way you act in your workouts is how you're going to act during theirs. And what you expect from yourself is what you're going to expect from them. You can't do the workouts for them, so they're gonna be counting on your spirit. They want to see that you're going to do for them what you do for yourself, and that's the actual strength part you'll need for this job. A person who is too weak to support himself cannot make a career out of supporting others. You'll need to show people the way, every day.

The final thing I want to talk about here is demographics. Don't get stuck only training people who are the most like you. I often attract young-to-middle-aged, able-bodied women who want stronger upper bodies. Great! But my gym has a huge variety of members. What about all the demographics who I don't represent? How can I show that I'm capable of enough range to train a senior, a man, or someone with a joint replacement? You'll use a phenomenon I call Demographics By Association. Whatever client you're working with at any given moment becomes part of your Demographics By Association. For example, if a seventy-year-old sees me training another seventy-year-old, the first one subconsciously associates me with her demographic. I'm like an adjunct to her. If a young male baseball player sees me training a young male football player, the former knows that I might understand his needs as well. Demographics By Association are an automatic advertisement for your skills. People feel like you'll be able to see them, because you see others who are like them.

My current client base spans eight decades of ages, is equal men and women, includes beginners and experts, able-bodied and disabled people, and ranges from students to CEOs. It's a blast. One supremely excellent part of this job is living in the thick of a very cool cross-section of society. When you have a full schedule, everyone, even the most unlikely clients, will fit into a Venn diagram of: people who are attracted to your teaching style; people who want your friendship; and people who want the fitness that you have to offer. It will be hard to judge which of these someone wants from you just by looking at them. So make a point to seek out conversations and offer advice to all kinds of people in the gym, not just the people who are the most obvious fit for you. You'll miss some extraordinary people and opportunities if you don't.

Most importantly, people want to know that you see them for who they are. If you can do this genuinely, you'll have as many clients as you want, for as long as you stay in the field.

<u>TL;DR</u>

1) Meet clients by having them assigned to you by sales staff, by teaching and subbing group exercise classes, by talking to people about themselves and their workouts, and by doing your own workouts in the middle of the gym. No matter how good the filter from sales is, you will largely be responsible for getting your own clients.

2) Never assume who would or would not be a good client for you. My first impressions have often been wrong. Give everyone a chance.

3) A good trainer understands their own strength and can communicate that to their client. Being the client is difficult. The workouts are hard, they feel watched—sometimes embarrassed—and they're not sure they can do what is being asked. A trainer's job is to make the client feel like they have a teammate, not a judge. Learn how to communicate mental strength as well as you communicate physical strength.

Chapter Five: Client Assessments (The Comp One)

After you've met a potential client and decided you like each other, it's time to get together for an assessment. Most gyms offer two free sessions with each membership: a body assessment and a movement assessment. (We always called them the Complimentary Session One and Complimentary Session Two. Abbreviated as Comp One and Comp Two.) The Comp One tends to look at the person's numbers: age, weight, body fat percentage, etc. The Comp Two usually takes place on the gym floor, where they can get a taste of your training style and whether they can see themselves training with you.

In this chapter, we're talking about the Comp One, the body assessment.

First thing to note: This appointment is generally stressful for most adults, especially women. It feels like an audition on the most personal and sensitive stage they've got: their own body. The majority of people are going to come in to the session wondering what you're gonna say about them. Even when people are fit, they're self-conscious about this appointment. And when they're not fit? They're preparing for an emotional bloodbath led by you, the gym's Hannibal Lecter, asking the most terrifying questions. *Hello, Clarice. How often do you currently exercise?*

What will you think of their body? Are they too out of shape to even start? What kind of pinching, prodding, measuring, weighing, and other humiliating tactics will you use? Is the whole thing just going to be a sales pitch? And scariest of all: Are they hopeless?

Given this fear, it's amazing and brave that people, especially women, agree to come in at all. Humanity's collective opinion of what a fit and healthy body should be might not seem like it's related to your personal assessments. But our societal view of bodies, weight, and physical abilities is something that's crushed nearly all of us at one point or another. If you want to connect with a new client quickly, you need to make an effort to understand what might be in their environmental history. All of us 90's kids spent the entire decade reading tabloids titled Best and Worst Beach Bodies, with "hideous" celebrity body parts circled in red. Bridget Jones was a blockbuster sensation movie starring Renée Zellweger, desperate to lose weight and get a man. The whole movie was one giant fat joke. Her weight? 136 pounds. Three pounds lighter than I am right now, writing this sentence as a size four.

By no means do 90's kids claim to be the only fucked-up generation. Look at what we've all had to internalize in the name of selling us a "better" body. The generations where women were told to stay home and brush their hair 100 times a day instead of exercising (silent generation). Where women were forbidden from doing sports and discouraged from sweating because it's gross (boomers). Where people lived in terror of eating absolutely anything with fat content (gen X). And where we collectively worshipped thinness so much that there was an entire fashion movement called "heroin-chic" (millennials). These histories still strongly affect the people who will come meet with you today.

The Zoomers are more inclusive of bodily sizes (we stan). But Gen Z has a different problem when it comes to nutrition and exercise. Every piece of advice they get about health comes in highly-targeted, manipulative, fifteen-second bites on TikTok.

Y'all. We gotta bring books back. There's no way of vetting whether the TikToker giving the advice has any qualifications, nor if that advice is backed by any research. Creating a video for views and shares means that nuance disappears, black-and-white opinions are made about grey topics, and difficult concepts get grossly oversimplified in order to make the point in forty-five seconds. Gen Zers and Millennials often come into the gym trying to set up random exercises they saw on Instagram, convinced it's going to instantly change their back pain (because, after all, that was the POV). Spoiler alert: it's not.

No matter who comes through your door, they're going to have some societal bodily baggage to deal with, and you'll want to figure out immediately what that baggage is, how you can work with it now, and hopefully how you can unravel it in the future.

Sadly, this isn't how gyms teach you to do an assessment.

Here's the assessment I was taught to do as a new trainer at a large corporate gym in 2008:

1. Get the person's name, age, and height. Take their weight by having them stand on our scale. Take their resting heart rate and blood pressure. Enter this info into our computer program.
2. Measure their chest, belly, upper arm, and thigh size with a measuring tape. Enter those measurements into the computer.
3. Use calipers (little pinchers) and my fingers to pinch and measure the amount of fat on the belly, tricep, and thigh. You're trying to get as much fat as you can between your fingers but not include muscle. Repeat a couple times to make sure you got accurate results. Enter those measurements.
4. Do a three-minute step test on a step with risers. Record their heart rate at the end and record how quickly their heart rate drops in the next minute. A heart rate that drops quickly upon resting is generally healthier than one that stays high for a long time.
5. Ask them to do as many pushups on the floor as they can.

Record.
6. Ask them to do as many sit-ups on the floor as they can.
Record.

That's it! In our gym's opinion, this was a perfect starting point for new clients. We would print out a few pages which contained their waist-to-hip ratio, their body fat percentage, BMI, and percentile ranking for cardio and strength for their age. I would review it with them, letting them know that the computer thinks they are a little bit fat and that their cardio sucks. They often left looking deflated, somber, or like their session went exactly how they feared. (I didn't pick up on these emotions at the time, but I sure can realize them now, looking back.)

This is still a normal assessment in plenty of gyms today. I don't remember when I started thinking this routine was bullshit but I performed these assessments on a LOT of people before I began second-guessing the whole thing. At the time, I was all, *ooh, this is good information. They should know these things about themselves.* I thought it was a neat computer program.

The assessment had other problems besides the calipers and measuring tape. The pushup test sucks. It's asking someone in regular work clothes, not warmed up, with no concept of their wrist, shoulder, or spinal health, to do a maximum pushup effort on the floor regardless of age or prior training. Like, what the fuck? I'm supposed to put stock in that data point? We think that's scientifically sound? As the bros would say, it's about as scientifically sound as deez nuts.

We had to measure sit-ups as well. The max number you can do in a minute. Sit-ups as a measure of fitness are largely useless. Doing them as fast as you can for a minute is certainly useless. A full sit-up requires the abs to do the crunch, and then a strong pull through the hip flexors to complete the sitting up part. So are we counting just the crunch part or does it have to be a full sit-up? The computer was measuring ab endurance, not hip flexor strength, so I would be fine with people doing crunches. But then, of course, there's a time issue. It takes much longer to complete a sit-up than a crunch. So are we doctoring the numbers here? WHAT IF THEY DO FIFTY CRUNCHES INSTEAD OF THIRTY SIT UPS? WHAT DOES THAT MEAN??? HOW CAN WE CONTINUE TRAINING WITH THIS CLOUD OF ABDOMINAL UNCERTAINTY HOVERING OVER US AT EVERY MOMENT?

(Cloud of Abdominal Uncertainty is going to be the name of my riveting memoir about life with gas.)

A three-minute step test is actually a fine introductory measure of cardiac ability. But without having ever seen the person move before, I couldn't have any idea of whether they were doing the test with me at a doable pace, a challenging pace, or a brutally fast pace for them. All three will give totally different results without any information on what a person's usual habits and abilities are. Do they always do cardio this fast or are they just trying to impress me in the moment? Are they purposely slowing down to make sure they can complete the whole time without embarrassing themselves? It was like asking someone to read a paragraph in Mandarin to determine their ability in world languages as a whole. It will technically give you a clue, but not a very useful one.

So these assessments were garbage, partly because the scientific rationale behind them was poor. But we need to talk about the real reason they were garbage, which took me way too long to figure it out and I'm hoping you'll get there much sooner.

This assessment protocol was secretly 100% fat-focused. On the printout that we would give people at the end, everything was written in red, and all of the results tied back to their weight, even the strength-testing results. The computer demanded to know: *Just how fat are you? Can you see by these three different measurements that you are fat? The poor results on this cardio test suggest that you might be fat, or at risk of becoming fat. If you weren't fat you could do more pushups. Your stomach fat is getting in the way of your sit-ups. Your BMI is a warning sign about being fat. Your waist-to-hip ratio is a signal that you have too much fat. Can you see how your body fat percentage is way over a healthy range? It's written in bold red scary lettering on this printout, that's how you can tell.*

It was brutal.

I'd love to write here that I was put off by this assessment because of how degrading it was. But it's not true. I was put off by this assessment because it told me nothing about the person's actual physical condition. I would get to our second complimentary session and feel like I was starting from scratch. Remember that the Comp Two is a sample workout with your new client. I'd be going into these workouts feeling totally unprepared. So this person can do thirty-two sit ups in a minute, ten pushups in a minute, and has a body fat percentage of 28%. Okay? What am I supposed to do with this information? Are we supposed to work on improving their pushup endurance? I've never even asked them if they *want* to learn a pushup.

I should have questioned my aggravation more deeply than that. At the time, I just wanted to learn how people's bodies moved so that I could train them, and I was irritated that the assessment didn't show me this. But if I'd taken it deeper, I could have figured out that the reason I was irritated wasn't the assessment at all. I was irritated because the message I'd always received—that being fat or thin was the most important body trait you could have—was ultimately pretty meaningless when it came to fitness.

The computer was supposed to tell me who was healthy and unhealthy and I was supposed to use that information to come up with an improvement program for them. If it told me someone was fat, I would wag my finger and look stern. If the computer told me someone was thin, I would praise them and tell them they were doing everything right. But then in the Comp Two, the first person might be moving heavy-ass weights and crushing tabatas on the bike, while the second person wasn't strong enough to lift the cat litter out of the car. So who was healthier? My unease (I now know) was stemming from being unable to ignore the evidence that a central belief of mine might not be correct.

But let's set this comprehensive reconstruction of a deeply-entrenched societal construct aside for one moment. This assessment protocol was simply bad for business. I can't believe my old employers didn't realize this sooner. Plenty of people never came back for a second session, even though it was free. It sounds unbelievable, but it seems like manually pinching people's skin between our fingers, measuring it with a stick, and giving them five printed pages of fat-shaming diagnosis didn't make them want to return for more.

Huh.

As it dawned on me that there could be a better way to evaluate people, I finally went to my boss and told him that I would no longer be doing the company-mandated assessments. I griped that I didn't feel comfortable doing them and that I didn't learn anything useful about the person and that I really just wanted to talk to them instead and would that be ok? I was nervous he would fire me if I didn't comply with the rules (a commentary on being a woman in the workplace), but instead he said, "Sure, that's fine."

That's it? I could have done this all along? Well, shit. Why didn't anyone tell me?

I consider this conversation one of the turning points in my training career. I stopped pinching people's fat and started asking them to tell me about their secret fitness dreams. We chatted about the injuries they had as a kid, the way they loved field hockey, and how they're jealous of their spouse being able to run 5k's all the time. I learned that they have rambunctious kids, or kids who live far away, or kids who have died. It's counterintuitive maybe, but seeing them do pushups and sit-ups didn't tell me anything about what they might be capable of in the gym. Hearing them talk about surviving grief, or light up when they said they wished they could run again but heard they were too old? Now THAT gave me something to go on. Because it's not a person's fat cells that tells me what they can do, it's their spirit and their history. Their drive, their determination, their interest in proving themselves. You show me that, and I'll know exactly what you can become in the gym.

Now when I meet with a client, we simply talk for forty-five minutes to an hour. I always start the same way. "Tell me about yourself. How did you end up here today?" and then we take it from there. If you're wondering how learning about someone's family can tell you about where to start their training programs, let me explain. Being a personal trainer requires excellent people skills. You need to be able to relate to them, fast, and you need to be able to read them, fast. Not just in the first session but in every session. What's happening in their life will affect their ability to perform any given workout and complete any given training block. Not many mothers of infants are going to be able to complete a three-month hypertrophy mesocycle. Not many law school grads are gonna be well-positioned to prepare for a marathon that's three months away when the bar exam is four months away.

So when you meet a new potential client, your first priority should be learning a little bit about them. Get their perspective of what health and fitness means to them, and ask how they see themselves relative to that perspective. If someone tells me their goal is to be healthier, I always say, "What does healthy mean to you?" If someone tells me they want to be stronger, I always say, "What makes you feel strong?" If someone says they want to feel better, I always ask, "What are you currently feeling badly about?"

Here are some questions that I always ask new clients, along with what their answers teach me. But as you establish yourself in the field, I am positive you will come up with your own list of questions and your own answers that you need to feel prepared to work with someone. And don't obsess over it. A natural conversation is much more important than running down a list of questions about goals and obstacles.

First, say hi, and ask how they're doing. Ask what brought them in to see you that day, especially if they mention they've been trying to get in shape for a long time. Why now? Why today? What changed? This answer needs to stay in your head as the lens through which you'll view all the other answers. Even if it's "I don't know," you know that they felt some kind of draw to come in now and not yesterday, so keep looking for it.

After that, some of these will help clarify the picture for you:

Did you do sports as a kid? How did that go?

This is always one of my first questions. It tells you if someone has an athletic background—no matter how long ago—and if they enjoyed it. It gives you an indication of the kind of exercise they enjoy: a former gymnast (absolutely no endurance, loves sprints) will have had very different sport experiences than a former cross-country runner (absolutely no lifting, loves endurance). Their opinion can have changed since then, obviously, but odds are good that they still love many aspects of their former sport. This will help you narrow down a place to begin with them.

You might also learn if they were bullied in sports or had a bad coaching experience. Things like this can affect their self-esteem in the gym and in their relationship with you. The instant someone suggests they had a questionable coaching, I try to find out what the issue was. We'll talk more about trust later, but your client will need reassurance (possibly subconscious reassurance) that your coaching is not going to reflect that fear or power struggle they previously experienced. And you wouldn't believe how many adults have deep trauma from childhood gym class.

Finally, this question is an easy entry into the injuries conversation. I consider all injuries and surgeries relevant, whether they happened yesterday or fifty years ago. Remember that the physical therapy compliance rate is about 15%. That means that 85% of injuries are never properly rehabbed to completion. Any injury can still be relevant decades later, so don't let people say, "Oh, I broke my leg when I was twenty but it's never been a problem." In many people, you'll notice that leg the minute they hit a lunge.

What do you do for work? Do you have a family? Do you live nearby? Etc.

Questions about their non-gym life will give you a more complete picture of the person sitting in front of you. Some information is practical for you to know (for example, their job and hours will indicate when they could be available to come see you), others are just because, again, you want to understand who you're working with. If they're single, if they have kids, if they're part of a marginalized community, if they can walk to the gym, etc. All of these factors inform a schedule and a relationship. You may bond over things you share in common, or you might hear something that piques your interest. If the conversation is interesting, let it go off course here for a bit.

Tell me about your injuries and medical history.

So I always lead this off by reminding them that I only need to know stuff that could affect us in the gym. That means:

- Injuries: broken bones, sprains, unresolved tendinopathies, etc.

- Surgeries: traumatic events, joint replacements, hernias, hysterectomies, etc.

- Family history: heart attacks, strokes, aneurysms, etc.

- Chronic illness: asthma, balance disorders, hearing/vision loss, depression, etc.

- Medications: beta blockers, anything for the heart, anything related to diabetes, etc.

The story I always tell about this is one of my clients who assured me she had absolutely no health history at all, and then had a seizure during one of our sessions. It scared the everliving shit out of me. When she came to, she was like, oh it's totally normal because I have epilepsy. I was like, MA'AM? When I asked you if there were any health conditions that could affect our workouts, freaking EPILEPSY is on the list, ok? Sheesh.

You'll hear about chronic injuries the most. The nagging shoulder, the back pain that surfaces and disappears without notice. Take note of them so that you can look for them yourself in your second session with the person.

If they've had a surgery you're not familiar with, ask them if they still have any restrictions from that surgery. Even if it were a long time ago, the answer could definitely be yes (fusions, reconstructions, some replacements). Do some research later on the surgery so you can understand what it was and how you can safely work with it in the gym.

What are you currently doing for exercise? Anything? It's alright if the answer is no.

This can be a touchy one, because anyone who isn't doing any exercise is often shy or embarrassed to admit it. So I lead off by trying to reassure them that I'm not trying to lecture them, I'm just looking for complete information. The answer is often no, which is ok! It's why they're sitting in front of you now. They're literally trying to make the exact change you're asking about, so don't blow out that tiny spark. If they say no, praise them for taking the step of meeting with you, which, as I said, is tough for people, and even tougher for newbies.

If they do exercise, sometimes they'll say something like, "Oh, no I don't do anything, I just walk a few days a week," or "No, just yoga." This is the perfect place to show them that you're not part of the toxic wellness industry. Walking is exercise! Yoga is exercise! Having a fitness habit of any kind is already a great thing! Don't let them discount the work they're already putting in. It's super important that they recognize that even their small efforts count.

This question will also fill in the picture that was begun by the childhood sports question. People will often say that they used to have a trainer, or used to lift before they had kids, or loved running for thirty years but started having knee pain, etc etc. Even if they're not exercising now, having an exercise history is critical for you to know. Again, you'll hear what they're experienced in, what they have liked doing for exercise in the past, and what they wish they could do again. And speaking of...

If you could do absolutely anything in fitness or sports, what would you want to be able to do? Don't think about injuries, age, ability, or time. What do you wish you could do?

I love this question. First, you get to know a little more about someone's inner dreams. Always a good way to bond. Second, it's an opportunity to show them that it's okay to have personal ambitions as an adult. People (especially young parents, who are hyper-focused on their kids' wellbeing) often think their own goals are stupid, selfish, unreachable, or worse, unimportant. This puts a huge barrier in front of training for anything. Third, they're literally gonna tell you right here where you should start your programming. So don't forget their answer.

I once met a 77-year-old man who told me he hadn't run in twenty-five years but always wished that he could do it again because he loved it so much as a youth. I asked him why he stopped, and he said it was because he was worried it was bad for him as he got older. I said, "Do you want to run again?" and he said, "Do you think I could?" and I said, "Absolutely 100% yes."

Now, this was in our first meeting. We were just sitting in chairs and I'd never seen him move other than walking into the room with me. So what gives me the confidence to promise this man something this big?

1) His walking and gait were totally normal, especially for age 77. No visible mobility concerns.

2) His entire face lit up when he talked about running. That kind of joy is difficult to interfere with. I knew if he loved it that much, any variation of running would probably make him happy. No need for sprints or marathons (although I'd never rule those out either). We could probably just do some short jogs, which would be quite safe.

3) I believe with my entire soul that if a human wants to do something, they can find a way to do it, and I'll be damned if I'm the person who tells them not to. I love to say yes.

After this meeting, we did a whole bunch of sessions where we took a look at his leg strength, single leg stances, balance, core control, and then I sprung it on him. On a bright fall day, we warmed up normally and then I said, "You ready to go for a run today?"

His eyes got so big.

"You think I'm ready?"

"I think you're ready."

We ran together next to the Charles River for many years, in all weather, him shuffling along, me doing a fast walk next to him. Talking about family, writing, education, solving the world's problems, solving each other's problems, cursing up a blue streak—he's my only client who swears more than I do. One of my all-time favorite training memories, one of his all-time favorite training memories. Neither of us would have had this if I'd said no, running seems like a bad idea at your age.

Say yes to people. Promise them that you will try your hardest to get them closer to what they want. Don't promise them what they want, because you don't have that much control. Promise them that you will try your hardest to get them as close as possible, and then keep that promise.

In the course of a normal conversation, you might deviate far from these topics and that's fine. Remember, you're trying to learn more about the person in front of you, so follow the conversation where they take it.

A note: people will share extremely personal stuff with you. I often open a session by telling them that I'll be asking a lot of personal questions and that they are free to give me as much or as little information as they want, including deciding not to answer. Relatedly, if they share something personal with you that you didn't ask about (they're going through a divorce, they're estranged from a child, they just got fired, they were previously incarcerated, etc), I will make a quick judgment call on whether I need to know more. Sometimes I will ask permission to know more ("Can I ask you more about that?"), sometimes I will simply say, "Oh, I am so sorry that you are going through that," and move on. In circumstances where I'm not sure but it seems relevant to training, I will ask questions specifically about what they have shared (e.g. "Are you living on your own while you settle the divorce?" [indicates stress levels, time availability, and also possibly a location closer to/further from the gym which affects scheduling]), but I will not ask extra questions about what they have not shared (e.g. "Do you have custody of the kids?").

Handling people's secrets and their fragile histories is something that you will be doing right from the beginning. They're already trusting you with their bodies, which, in and of itself, is highly personal. It won't be long before they trust you with their personal lives as well. Your client should never, ever feel like you're going to abuse or disregard the information they're giving you. I'm extremely light-hearted during workouts, sarcastic and always making jokes and gently teasing people. But I never do that when they're sharing difficult stuff, and it's important to be able to recognize the time and place for each.

I've definitely made mistakes in navigating some super private conversations. A client of mine (fortunately this was not a first session, we had already trained for years), who deeply wanted another baby, was joyfully pregnant. She confided to me one day during a session that they had just learned that the fetus had a number of unfixable problems. We talked a bit, and I suddenly asked her if she was going to get an abortion. Why on earth I asked this question, no one will ever know. I'm still ashamed by it. She burst into tears, because of course she did. Not only none of my business, but how dare I ask her this when I knew full well that she was so, so happy to be pregnant again? Ugh. I wrote her an email to apologize later that night. Normally I would apologize face-to-face, but it was such a sensitive topic, I didn't want it to interfere with her next workout as well. She was kind in accepting my apology, and she did ultimately have a beautiful second child later on. But wow was that a mistake.

More than anything, become great at listening. Give people a safe space to share what's on their mind, right from the first session. They might ask for your advice or opinion, but lots of times they don't. Don't offer it unless they specifically want it. Just listen, and your client will begin trusting you immediately.

The last thing I do in an assessment is give clients a little bit of insight into my own background and training style. People want to know about you, too. They want to know what to expect from you and your sessions so they can be prepared. Do you lift heavy weights? Are you a cardio queen? Trainers are always informed by what they like to do themselves, no matter how hard we might try to avoid this. I tell them that I'm a specialist in bodyweight conditioning because of my gymnastics, and that I like to see them move around before making any decisions on the best place to start our work. If I said that I'm a bodybuilder, it would give the client a completely different impression about what I value and teach. Not better or worse, but completely different.

I also tell them what they can expect from their next appointment, which is a full workout. If I can tell that they're nervous about it, I'll spend a little extra time explaining the format and what I'll be looking for from them. Then, towards the end of the Comp One, I'll check in on whether they might be interested in doing some regular personal training. It's not a sales pitch (which I tell them immediately), it's a preparation question. Knowing whether they plan to work with you will affect how you run their second session. (Tell them this!) If they don't plan to work with you again, then you'll have one hour to teach them as much useful information as you can. In this case, I would organize the Comp Two as a general overview, hitting the biggest issues and giving them some tools to tackle those issues on their own.

If they do plan to work with you at least a few more times, then I'll treat their second session as day one of a program. We'll still do the general overview, but anything that sticks out as an issue I will immediately start figuring out how to program it over the next eight weeks or whatever. You can get a lot more specific in the Comp Two if you know you're going to have some time to work on it with your client.

As a last note, ALL of this hour should be spent hyping your client. The more you talk, the more excited they should get. By the end of it, they should be wishing that their next workout were starting immediately.

Don't be fake.

Do not make promises you can't keep.

Do not sell tickets to the supermodel body hallowed grounds.

Do be genuinely excited that your new client is there, taking steps towards change, trusting you to help them on the way, and recognize aloud that a brilliant new partnership is being formed as you speak. If you're excited to work with them, they're gonna be excited to work with you. People have such high hopes about adding fitness to their lives, but those hopes are paper thin in the beginning. They've been disappointed before. You want to give those hopes a little bit more substance, something real for your new client to be able to grab onto. That real thing is your excitement, energy, and belief in them.

Lastly, book their second session while they're still there in the room with you. Don't let them leave without doing this unless you absolutely have to.

That's it! You've made it through the first assessment. You know their background, their medical history, their dreams and lofty goals, and gotten them excited about moving forward. Now it's time to give your new potential client their first workout. This is where you'll solidify the fact that you offer a ton of cool shit—way more valuable than the price being charged—and that they're ready to truly benefit from that cool shit.

Get ready for the fun part; here comes the Comp Two.

TL;DR:

1) Learn everything you can about a new potential client. Make the effort to learn their name, spell, and pronounce it correctly. (You wouldn't believe how many people do not do this.) Find out about their life, in and out of sports. Remember these details.

2) Don't treat client assessments like a sale. You're not there to sell to them, you're there to meet them and find out how you can help them. If they want your help, they'll buy it.

3) When people tell you what they want at the gym, help them get it. Don't tell them it's unrealistic, inappropriate for their age, or anything else. My 92-year-old client once wanted to take boxing lessons. We got her boxing lessons. Do not take away the things that people want. Whether they should have it or not is none of your business.

Chapter Six: Client Assessments (The Comp Two)

The Comp Two—your first workout with a new client—is one of my favorite parts of being a personal trainer. I get SO excited to have someone new in my hands, and they're excited to be in my hands too. (Insert joke in three, two...) Even if you only have one hour together and they're never gonna train with you again, you have an opportunity to teach them something they can use forever. Not many jobs offer that kind of opportunity at any point, and you'll have it all the time. I love seeing potential in people, and Comp Twos are ALL about potential.

But when I first started as a trainer? Shit. I didn't have a single clue about how to run a Comp Two. I ran some really bad ones. Put some people at risk with too much intensity. Didn't start with the right exercises. Didn't home in on the right problems. Thought it was my job to make someone sore AF so they'd be blown away by how great I am at training. Boo, hiss. *Throws tomatoes at my novice trainer self* And it wasn't just my Comp Twos that were bad either. I *wish* the only bad workout I've taken people through was the first one. I'm going to tell you about a few instances where I really fucked things up; one with a new client, one with a regular client, and one in a group class. Even though only one of these was in a Comp Two specifically, all of them could have been prevented with better education about what a Comp Two is and does.

The purpose of a Comp Two is to get as much baseline info as possible about the person in front of you, in just one hour. You then use that info for everything that follows, from their next workout to their next five years of workouts. It's a skeleton of their future workout plan. Understanding the Comp Two structure gives you three things.

First, the starting point for a new client. If they're trying to improve their running, the Comp Two will show you whether the biggest issue is their hip extension, their uneven core mechanics, or their weak feet and ankles. Since you don't have time to work on everything all at once, you've got to prioritize. The Comp Two shows you the order of priority.

Second, it gives you a base for every client, which you can refer to at any time that you need guidance. No matter how long you've worked together, you will always be able to return to what you learned in the Comp Two and use that for your next bout of programming with that client. If you're getting lost in exercise selection, or if your client wants to shake things up, don't just randomly select new things for them to try. Go back to what you learned in your Comp Two and pick up from there.

Third, it will make you a much better group fitness instructor. Being a whiz at a Comp Two will let you evaluate a group class full of strangers in just a few minutes with just a few movements. The more quickly you can understand how a person's body moves, the more quickly you'll be able to assign anyone an appropriate level of work.

In the beginning, I couldn't do any of these things. In Mia Of The Past's defense, I just didn't know any better. (This goes back to my ongoing plea for more thorough education for trainers.) When I was a new trainer, my boss said to me, regarding the Comp Two, "Just put them through a workout." Well sure, I could do that. Unfortunately, the only experience I had to draw on for this was my background in gymnastics. This gave me two starting points for training other people, one good and one bad. The good one: my knowledge of biomechanics. You can't be bad at biomechanics when you've spent a lifetime studying one of the most complicated sports up close and personal. Gymnastics is a potent cocktail of angular momentum, acceleration, and spring constants. So I naturally understood physics and could easily notice and correct detrimental movement patterns.

This was all a good thing.

But it was a bad starting point too. Being a gymnast meant that my knowledge of the appropriate workout level for the average person was terrible. It was normal for me to aggressively condition through the first hour of a five-hour practice because gymnastics coaches are mentally ill. I'd only ever seen people do insanely hard workouts. I thought that's how workouts were always supposed to be for everyone.

This was a bad thing.

Gymnastics conditioning is intense, to say the least. Sprints, rope climbs, leg lifts, rebounding box jumps, pull-ups, skin-the-cats, bear crawls, alligator pushups. Conditioning like this before practice was completely normal. The part that really set me up badly for real life is that all the gymnasts I ever knew trained like this. This kind of intensity isn't saved for elites like Simone Biles and Aly Raisman. It's just how gymnasts train, no matter what future they may or may not have in the sport. So when I saw so many types of people—talented, untalented, old, young, high-level, low-level—doing these sorts of workouts, it was natural for me to think that ALL types of people should be doing these workouts. And why not? Gymnasts are strong as fuck. Why would that be a bad thing to encourage?

I was delighted to bring that style of exercise to my unsuspecting clients. I just didn't realize that basic gymnastic fitness is not representative of basic general population fitness. And let's just say, they were...less delighted.

This showed up first in my Comp Twos. Not only was my standard for exercise already extremely high, but I used to actively try and give people a wicked workout in our first session. I did this to prove to them that they would work harder with me than without me. Those early sessions weren't Comp Twos, they were third-degree manslaughter. And trying to kill people can go wrong. One man was still sore, ten days later. Ten days! He could have traveled to the International Space Station three times while he was healing. Way too long to be sore, totally inappropriate training by me. Another client that I trained for the first time was so sore the next couple days that she booked a doctor's appointment because she thought something was wrong. At the time I scoffed like, girl, please. Learn what sore muscles are. You're fine. But as time went on and I became a better trainer, I realized that I had left her in so much pain that she wanted medical attention. And I thought that was a HER problem? Please. That was 100% a me problem.

Pro tip: Don't murder your clients! ANYONE can make someone else sore. Go do five hundred burpees. You'll be sore, but that doesn't mean you got a productive workout. Sore isn't usually a problem, but it's also not a great measure of anything. You'll always have time to give your clients increasingly harder workouts. The first workout ain't it. Show them that you know what you're talking about and they'll hire you, no death and destruction needed.

Great Comp Two knowledge also helps you keep your client programming targeted and fresh, long after their first workout is over. I was once giving a workout to Nancy, a sixty-year-old regular client whom I had been training for a while. We got along great, and she was willing to try anything in her workouts, which I loved. But one day, I decided she needed some more pizzazz in her workouts. After racking my brain before her session, I knew just what I wanted to assign. I dragged a twelve-inch plyo box over to her and said, "OK, time for box jumps."

She gamely moved over to stand in front of the box.

I said, "No, no. Turn around. We're going backwards."

Backwards box jumps are a common drill in gymnastics. You stand with your back to the box, do a two-leg backwards jump onto it, hop back down to the ground, and immediately rebound back up again. It helps you learn a quick punch into a back flip.

I can't believe I have to write this sentence, but this grandmother didn't actually need to be doing drills for faster back flips. This never occurred to me. I just knew it was a common plyometric move done by everyone I knew, and she was good at regular box jumps. So in my search for pizzazz, I figured we could spice them up.

"I don't think I can do that," she said.

"Of course you can. I've seen you jump."

"No, I don't think I can do it."

"You definitely can. Give it a try."

"I'm scared."

"You're good."

She moved slowly to the block, and turned her back to it.

"Perfect. Go ahead. Just jump right up. You got it."

She stood there for an eternity. And then, all of a sudden, she burst into tears and said, "Please, Mia, I'm so scared of trying this. I can't do it." I'm talking face-buried-in-her-hands, weeping. The other gym-goers turned to stare.

I immediately felt awful, told her it was no problem, put the box away, and we moved on. So at least I recognized the issue immediately and fixed it. But it should never have happened. Readers, I know you're new, but FYI you're not supposed to pressure your client so much that they start sobbing uncontrollably. Kind of frowned upon. You're also not supposed to assign random exercises just because they pop into your head. When you need a change with a client, you go back to your Comp Two and choose another area of weakness which needs improvement. If I truly wanted Nancy to work on moving backwards plyometrically (a useful skill even if you aren't backflipping), we could have changed the set in plenty of ways: stepping backwards onto the box instead of jumping; hopping backwards on flat ground; or backpedaling. Learn how to find another option for when these situations come up. As an aside, from the minute you begin working with a client, you should be able to substitute an exercise immediately if things aren't going well. Even if the one you chose seems fine to you. If your client is terrified, find another way. There's always another way.

Comp Twos also help you teach better group fitness classes. The first class I ever taught was a substitution for a PIT class—Power Interval Training. Fuck yeah. I was nervous to teach group exercise classes in general, but I knew I could teach that one. Power intervals are a gymnast's bread and butter.

About twenty minutes into class, one of my attendees, who is still a friend to this day, pulled me aside and quietly said, "Mia...this class is EXTREMELY difficult. I think it's too much for them."

I was stunned. I had come up with a program that was about half of what a normal conditioning session for our gymnastics team would be. I was sure it would be fine. I looked around at this group of middle-aged men and women, whom I had never met, doing long-duration sprints in the park combined with box jumps on benches, all with their stiff knees and slow feet. Everyone was doubled over, panting, and beet red. I did what any responsible human would do.

"Eh. They'll be fine," I said.

Looking back on it now, he was absolutely right. It was a crazy class to give to a group of people I'd never met. Did I mention it was 1pm in the middle of summer? I hadn't even considered the heat, since I didn't realize that we weren't all used to training in a pizza oven shaped like a gymnastics gym. With more Comp Two experience, I could have quickly evaluated this group and created an appropriate workout for the conditions. It might have still been sprints and jumps, but it would have been shorter duration work, longer rest, and not lasted for an entire hour. Good lord. I'm grateful that I didn't give anyone heatstroke.

As I've said, you're going to make mistakes as a trainer. These three experiences taught me how to do a better job evaluating the people in front of me, and to think more carefully about programming their workouts so that they fit. You'll make mistakes when you're new, and you'll make them when you're experienced. You're gonna realize one day that you've been teaching things that aren't scientifically sound, or things that you were never qualified to teach in the first place, or things that you don't personally believe in anymore. For example, a lot of trainers start to recognize that advanced hypertrophy techniques and daily metcons are pretty damaging to a body. You get strong and fit AF, but at a huge potential cost. As trainers begin understanding the concept of lifelong fitness, they usually start to think that maybe that cost needs to be prorated a bit, and their workouts change.

If you used to teach stuff that you don't teach anymore, great! That's how science is supposed to work. If you don't change your mind about things as you become more educated, get the fuck out of this field and every field. Exercise science is imprecise and always changing, and the human body is one of the most difficult subjects in the world to study. You *should* be changing your mind as new science and new research emerges (and when you come across old stuff that you haven't seen before). I look back on lots of sessions and clients and classes and wish that I knew then what I know now, because I could have done better for them.

Still, that's okay! Surgeons and chiropractors and massage therapists feel the same way. Caring for another living human is difficult work and you won't always get it right. As long as you are taking it seriously, and keeping your clients safe to the best of your ability, that's the most important thing. I know that Mia In The Past did the best she could. But I wish that I'd had a mentor to make the learning process easier.

Like I'm gonna do for you right now.

New trainers need to be taught how to evaluate a new client's physical abilities. It's not easy. You don't know a single thing about them. How do you know where to start safely? Is it just guessing?

A little bit, yes. The first workout will always be trial and error because you have no idea what their body can and cannot do. Make an educated guess about the first few movements you ask for and then start tailoring their exercises from there.

For me, the Comp Two always starts identically, but never finishes the same way as any other person's Comp Two. I'll teach you how I start most of the time, and then give you some guidance for how to use the information you learn. And remember, if your client has pain at any point, double check that they have seen someone about it. You are not qualified to treat injuries.

The basics of movement are squat and hinge (lower body), push and pull (upper body), rotate and balance (central body). Nearly all of the infinite exercises on the planet will fit into one of these categories. So when I'm evaluating a new client, I try to assess all of them, and I assess them in three ways. Mobility, Strength, and Speed. These build on each other, so mobility is the foundation. You cannot have good strength unless you have good mobility. Following that, you cannot be fast if you are not strong. In the Comp Two, mobility assessment is my priority. Simply, can they squat or can't they? If they can squat, I'll know it's safe to load with weight (how much weight will be determined down the road). If they can squat with weight, I know it's safe to add speed via plyometrics, dynamic kettlebell work, or Olympic lifts. But you only have an hour, so assessing mobility is the priority.

Pay close attention during the Comp Two (or take notes), because these six basic skills are very different. In the end, you'll find one that's strongest and one that's weakest, and that's how you'll know where to start your client's future program.

Unless my client has an unusual disability of some kind, or they've told me about a fresh injury, my first workouts will assess the following exercises. You can see videos of all of them on my Instagram page. The essential questions to answer about everything in your client's body are: Does it move at all? Then, does it move well? And then, could it move fast?

• Squats

Question one: can they perform some version of sitting down and standing back up again, which is the most basic human movement? I always have them sit and stand from a block first; a high one if they're beginner, a low one if they're advanced. If the block is easy, I take it away and ask for a regular bodyweight squat. I always ask them to go as low as they can, because I'm an ass-to-grass kind of girl. (Thank you, Malden, Massachusetts.) Most people can't go ass-to-grass, so then I ask them to hold at their lowest point of a squat and then tell me what's preventing them from going lower.

Here you're looking for:

○ **Ankle mobility.** If their dorsiflexion is bad, they'll tell you that they're gonna fall backwards if they go lower.

○ **Spine movement.** If they can't flex (round) their lowest spine while squatting, they'll just keep folding forward at the hips, dropping their chest more and more towards the floor. *(Yes, with a heavy squat you want to limit spinal flexion and extension during the lift. But for testing purposes, the fact that they *can't* round is important for you to know. Very, very few people can biomechanically sit down in an ass-to-grass squat with a perfectly flat, motionless spine. If you watch great squatters, you'll see that even the big guns have a bit of spinal movement as they go.)* If your client can't extend their spine, they'll do the opposite of above: rounding more and more as they lower down. Often these people can do ass-to-grass but they end up curled like a shrimp at the bottom.

○ **Knees.** If people have sore knees, they'll usually tell you here, but knee pain rarely prevents someone from physically being able to squat. They just don't *like* doing it because it hurts. A movement restriction and pain are two different things. (i.e. poor ankle mobility absolutely prevents someone from physically being able to squat. It's like a brick wall in the legs. Knee pain isn't usually like this.) If they have knee pain, check in to make sure they've seen a doctor or physical therapist about it.

○ **Overall leg strength.** Whatever their lowest squat point is, can they stand up out of it easily? Or do they struggle, sway, shift, squirm, or use their hands to get back up again? A struggle to come back up is almost always either a quad strength problem (they drop their chest far forward to stand), or a hip/glute strength problem (their knees wobble in and out like they're dancing the Cupid Shuffle).

If they can go ass-to-grass and come back up with no issues? Or if they can go ass-to-block and stand up with no issues? I'll make sure they can do ten or fifteen consistent reps, and then I'll know what range of motion I can safely load in future sessions.

• Lunges

I use my best judgement for which kind of lunge to begin with. If they're already athletic and not a fall risk, I will have them try a forward and backward lunge walk down the floor. If they're not super athletic but not a fall risk, I'll have them try lunges in place (forwards or backwards is fine). If they are a fall risk, or if they're a total beginner, I'll have them hold onto a railing or a Smith rack and show me some supported lunges. If they're comfortable lunging with the bar, then I'll bring them into an open space and see what happens when we freeball it. (Metaphorically speaking.)

Here you're looking for:

◦ **Stability.** Do they lose balance immediately? On both sides or just one side? This is often a dynamic core strength problem. Dynamic core strength requires strong feet and a midsection that braces before and throughout a movement.

◦ **Alignment of joints.** Do their knees cave in towards each other as they drop down in the lunge? A sign of hip/glute weakness.

○ **Strength.** Can they go all the way down and up? If the front knee straightens early on the way up, so their butt kicks backwards and their chest drops, this is likely a quad strength problem. If they shove forward into the knee to stand up, this is likely a butt and hamstring problem.

○ **Mobility.** Do their hips, knees, ankles, and toes all move comfortably into flexion or is something getting stuck on the way? A surprising number of people will tell you that it's the toes of the back foot which are preventing them from going down further. Toes that can't move comfortably into flexion are going to cause major problems in hikers/runners/stair climbers. Their calves, Achilles, and plantar fascia will be in peril. Do not ignore it if someone says they're feeling restricted in their toes/big toe, especially if that's the main restriction.

○ **Posture.** Can they keep their chest up through the whole range of motion or does it fall forward? An inability to be upright at the bottom of the lunge with the back hip extended shows a posterior chain problem; the butt, hamstrings, and lower back either can't get into extension, or can't locate any strength there. This person will almost always complain about super tight quads as well.

• Single-leg Romanian deadlifts

(also part of the balance portion of the program)

SLRDLs are one of my top-three favorite exercises. In sixteen years of training, I still do them all the time with nearly all my clients. They're useful, easily scaled, easy to load, and great for training multiple components: balance, core, hips, feet, the entire posterior chain, and the act of hinging itself.

Here you're looking for:

◦ **Balance.** Can they stand on one leg, keep a flat back, and hinge down to touch their knee, shin, foot, or floor, and come back up again on one leg without falling? If they keep touching their free foot to the floor, pay attention to the point where this happens. At the top when they're vertical? Hip strength issue. At the bottom when they're lowest? Hamstring weakness. On the way down? Poor hinging technique. On the way up? Posterior chain doesn't know how to engage as one unit.

◦ **Squareness.** Can they reach down without either rounding their back or losing their horizontal hip line? In other words, if someone is balanced on their right leg, you're looking to see if their left hip tilts and rises or if it stays square with the right hip. A rising left hip would indicate weakness in the hip adductors and abductors. A rounded back indicates either a lack of spinal extension ability, poor end-range hip flexion, weak hamstrings, or all of the above. (Those things often go together.)

◦ **Hinge.** Can they show a proper hinge? You should be able to see their bodyweight shift backwards into the butt and hamstrings immediately upon starting the descent. Their pelvis should rotate on top of the standing femur, closing the front angle of the hip, and the spine shouldn't move. Some people can take this hinge all the way to floor, but not most people. You don't have to be able to touch the floor to make this a valuable exercise. Almost all ranges of motion here are work, so only train your client through a clean hinge and don't force extra ROM they don't have. Make sure they stay back in the butt and hams on the way up again. Many people subtly shift forward at the turnaround point. A shift forward removes tension from the posterior chain and places it into the quads instead. The knee should be softly bent throughout a SLRDL, but if you see it bend more on the way up, that's a sure sign of the quad taking over for the posterior chain. (Requiring someone to keep their butt in contact with the wall behind them is a great tool for teaching this.)

• Pushups

This is a super interesting one. You're testing any version of a pushup, from hands on the wall to hands on the floor. I just use my best guess for starting point, but remember it's always better to start too easy and make it harder than the other way around. I will start most people by putting their hands on a plyo box and moving down as needed.

Here you're looking for:

◦ **Strength.** Can they touch their chest to the surface their hands are on and push back up again without breaking a straight body line? If no, then one of two things are in play here: either lack of strength or *perceived* lack of strength. Unfortunately, upper body training is so uncommon for many people—especially women—that the minute an upper body exercise feels even the slightest bit hard, they collapse. They're not used to stress being put through their arms in the same way that we are used to it with our legs. A perceived lack of strength is a completely different problem than an actual lack of strength.

How can you tell the difference? Take a look at the body shape of the negative (the part of the pushup movement that goes downwards, with gravity). People with an actual lack of strength will struggle with the negative. Their hips will drop immediately, the chest will sag, their head will sag, and their knees might bend too. If they're struggling on the way down, they'll struggle on the way up.

But people with a perceived lack of strength don't do this. They'll keep a straight body line all the way until their chest touches the surface their hands are on. Only then will they collapse, lose the body line, or otherwise let you know that they can't push back up. These are the people whose arms simply need to spend more time in that low, stressful position. Don't get me wrong: they will protest the shit out of you. They will tell you a thousand times that they can't do it because they're too weak. But they're only half right. They can't do it, but it's not because they're too weak. It's because they don't yet know how to generate the necessary strength. Trust me: if they can lower down cleanly, then they're strong enough to push up again.

◦ **Mobility.** Can they keep their head and neck lifted instead of dropping their nose/forehead towards the floor? Do both shoulder blades retract evenly as they move down, and protract as they move up? Do they shrug like crazy? Do their elbows and wrists bear their weight without issue?

◦ **Endurance.** They can do one good pushup but can they do six? Twelve? Twenty? Many people have three or four great pushups and then fall apart. This is an endurance problem, not a strength problem.

◦ **Core.** This falls under the strength category above but bears repeating. Their ab, back, and pelvic muscles should be able to control the body line throughout the movement. Plenty of people with strong arms breezing through pushups have a jacked-up midsection that's just kind of along for the ride. You can identify this by how their core doesn't keep the shoulders and hips connected when they're pushupping. Usually the hips are dropped well below the level of the shoulders.

• Pull-ups

I test pull-ups with my kids and with my ninety-year olds. Just like the pushups, you'll have to decide an appropriate place to start your client's pull-ups. I nearly always start on a Smith rack doing body rows of some kind. A beginner will be mostly standing up. A moderate will be parallel to the ground, hips up, feet flat on the floor, knees bent. An expert would go right onto a bar for a traditional pull-up.

Here you're looking for:

◦ **Strength.** Can they hang comfortably? If no, raise their body row up a little more vertically. Feeling like their hands are going to slip off the bar is terrifying for them and unhelpful for you. Next, can they touch their chest to the bar with a straight body? Check the movement: are their shoulder blades retracting? Is their thoracic spine extending? Collarbones spreading apart? Or, are they shrugging like crazy, hunching and rounding in order to force their sternum to touch the bar? And can they lower back down to the start position with control?

○ **Mobility.** In this case, mobility goes right alongside strength and it can be hard to determine which is the problem. Are they rounding towards the bar because their pullers are weak? Or are their rounding towards the bar because their t-spine doesn't extend enough to allow a straight body? You'll determine the answer by checking their t-spine for extension in another exercise.

○ **Scapular movement.** This also goes alongside strength but deserves its own category. To me, this is the most important thing to note. It can be tricky, because people are wonderful at creating compensations. Do the shoulders/shoulder blades retract and depress as the person pulls or do they shrug up and forward towards their ears as they pull? The shrug suggests: poor mid/lower trap strength, poor rhomboids/scap retractor strength, an inability to access the lats, and possibly poor spinal extension. The good news for you is that nearly all of these are likely to be true if the person is showing a hard shrug, so you can just work on all of them concurrently. Keep looking: do their shoulder blades start the movement or do their elbows start the movement? If the elbows are the first thing to pull, you know that the scapular patterning is dead wrong, even if they ultimately do pull down and back by the time the person reaches the top of the pull-up. Shoulder blades are the base of every single arm movement on this planet. If they do not move or brace first, something is not correct.

• Rotations

Rotation technically applies to all the joints, but in this circumstance I'm talking about spinal rotation on the transverse plane, hip rotation, and shoulder rotation. Everything we've done so far has been on the sagittal plane, but you need to evaluate your client in three dimensions. Rotation is pretty easy to look at: can they turn or no? For spinal rotation, I usually start seated, arms crossed across the chest, because it blocks the hips from compensating. Have them turn in each direction as far as they can without shifting any weight in their butt bones.

Here you're looking for:

○ **Mobility.** A healthy spine should be able to rotate at least forty-five degrees in each direction while seated. Does it look like a nice spiral up the spine, or does it look like one giant chunk? In a perfect world, each vertebral joint adds to the rotation individually. The movement should reflect that. If it looks stiff, or like a chunk of torso turning on a chunk of hips, then some spinal segmentation drills should go on the menu. (Chunk Of Torso Chunk Of Hips is gonna be the name of my all-girl heavy metal band.)

○ **Strength.** If they have good rotational range of motion, can they take a weight through that same range of motion or does it stop much sooner? I will use an exercise band to test this. Sometimes spines can rotate great without resistance, but the minute you add a light band it's like slamming into a wall.

° **Hip rotation.** Hip internal and external rotation are critical movements, both for the hips themselves, and also in relation to back pain, knee pain, and foot pain. You can test these in various 90-90 positions if your client can get there, or in exercises like airplanes and hip CARS.

° **Shoulder rotation.** Again, shoulder internal and external rotation are critical movements. The vast majority of chronic shoulder injuries can be traced to weak rotator cuffs. There are a thousand ways to evaluate this. Start easy (like 90-degree IR and ER) and look for any obvious glitches before trying more difficult ones (like prone ER on the floor or anything with a long arc).

• Balances

Lastly, I look at balance. Have them take their shoes off. I've already started testing them with the single-leg Romanian deadlifts. If they've already shown me a full-range-of-motion SLRDL with great balance, I move them right into single-leg calf raises without holding on. (These are the holy grail of balance.) If they haven't shown me a SLRDL with great balance, I'll regress a bit. We will try standing on one foot or in tandem stance, and, if it seems safe, test these with eyes closed. Finally, I'll usually try some marching in place with a kettlebell in just one hand, suitcase-style. This will show you a few things: their anti-flexion/anti-rotation abilities, their balance with a lopsided weight, and their core endurance while standing.

Here you're looking for:

○ **Posture.** A body that's properly standing on one foot should be vertical, with the standing hip pushed out slightly past the body's midline. This will put the center of mass over the arch of the foot. Many, many people will balance with their shoulders leaned over to the side instead of their hip pushed out to the side, so they're tilted on an angle. This indicates either poor hip strength or poor hip function, something for you to determine as you go.

○ **Feet.** What is their foot doing while balancing? It's normal and necessary for the foot and ankle to make micro-adjustments in order to balance everything that's on top. People always think they're supposed to stand there like stone, but that's not true. I always compare it to balancing a baseball bat on your palm. Your hand will move beneath the bat in order to compensate for any changes happening up top. It's fine for the foot to make adjustments. However, it should stay planted atop all three arches while making those adjustments.

(A review: there are three arches of the foot, not just one. The medial arch, which runs from the big toe knuckle to the heel; the longitudinal arch, which runs pinky toe to heel; and the transverse arch, which runs horizontally underneath the ball of the foot. They make a triangle.) You're looking for your client to be balancing with all five toes flat (not curled or clutching), the entire ball of the foot level, and the center of the heel on the floor. This will naturally set their weight in the center of that arched triangle. The most common mistake is to let the big toe knuckle peel up while trying to

balance, so the person's weight is shifted on the outside edge of their foot. Big toe knuckle must stay flat.

This is a critical balance test: When a body is balancing properly, there should be strength on the diagonal between the medial ball of the foot and the outer hip. When glute med and glute min are not strong enough (or poorly patterned), and/or when the foot is too weak to dissociate itself from the ankle and hold itself flat, you'll see the client's foot constantly rolling over the pinky side. Their body is shifting ALL of the weight sideways because their hip and foot can't provide support without the entire center of mass moving.

A proper balance should feel the big toe knuckle pressing down firmly into the floor, carrying that strength up the leg to the outer hip, which pushes out sideways (away from the big toe), and then up another diagonal from the hip to the opposite shoulder. Again, you can find videos of this on my Instagram page.

○ **Endurance.** Have them stay balanced for a while. What is getting tired? Most people will say their calf/ankle stabilizers, which is fine although they shouldn't be screaming. Some will say the bottom of their foot gets tired fast, which is a sign of poor intrinsic foot muscles. Encourage your clients to spend more time barefoot at home. If the lateral hip is what's getting tired, then you know you'll need a whole glute med improvement plan in place ASAP.

So that's the framework I always intend to use for a Comp Two: squats, lunges, hinges, SLRDLs, pushups, pull-ups, rotations, and balance. This whole process should take about an hour and give you TONS of information about your client's body. For some people, we don't finish them all, which is fine. For others, we fly through and I can add more exercises.

If I've got time, I might also look at someone's glute bridges, side planks, and calf raises (I always look at calf raises if the person is a runner or jumper). I might look at an advanced athlete's jumping, running, and single-leg squats. You don't need to do sets or count reps super carefully at this part of the game. Your priority is to look at the movement quality. The places with poor movement quality are going to be your starting points. If there are several poor movements, start by addressing the ones that most influence your client's goals.

These assessments will point you in the right directions to start. But don't worry: you'll have plenty of trial and error ahead of you. Just remember than any client will have many good starting points (no one ever has just one problem), and they will benefit from you improving any of them. So don't stress too much about finding the exact right exercise all the time. The more you get to know your client, the easier it will get to create their program.

And, yes, I really do use these same exercises for almost everyone. I'd use them on a ninety-year-old who wants to be able to get in and out of a car, and I'd use them on a lifter who's trying to crack a 500-pound deadlift. There will be plenty of time down the road to look at their heavy deadlift. For now, go bodyweight. The point of using simple bodyweight exercises to evaluate people is that you can see their base movement patterns clearly. If they can't hinge a single-leg deadlift correctly, they're not hinging 500 pounds correctly either. Anything that shows up in an easy exercise will show up times a thousand in a difficult one.

Here's a story. I trained a guy with a 700-ish pound squat for a while. He was starting to have all kinds of plateaus, most of them related to pain and stiffness. He couldn't get the needle to move any further and was looking for help from someone who wouldn't just program more and more weight for him. While some of that stiffness is bound to occur when you're lifting small elephants, it's always worth regressing to the baseline to double-check. When I tested his single-leg squat, he couldn't sit down cleanly to an eighteen-inch box and stand up again. On either leg. There was absolutely no stability anywhere. I couldn't believe he was able to lift so much weight with so many energy leaks. I knew exactly what would happen if he focused on different work for a while. After a solid program of bodyweight conditioning with me to complement his lifting, he texted me that he had just hit 750 pounds and it felt easy. It was awesome to watch, and a good lesson. When your clients are struggling, always go back to basics first, to look for what might have been missed on the way.

I have another client who loves to run. When we first met, I asked him to show me his single-leg calf raise and he said, "Sure, just know that I broke this foot a couple years ago so it's not as strong as the other one." That's already a giant red flag. But when he did his calf raise, his whole ankle fell out laterally on every rep. He couldn't correct it. If I asked him to force his ankle into a straight line, he couldn't lift a quarter inch off the ground. Not one quarter of an inch. There aren't too many guarantees in the human body but this is one of them: If this man cannot do a calf raise while standing in place, holding on for balance, without his ankle falling out sideways, then his ankle is falling out sideways on every single running step he takes. Guaranteed. Not only does it make his running inefficient, but is very likely to turn into a chronic injury somewhere else: peroneals, stress fractures, knee issues, back pain.

Instead of trying to clean up his stride and do a bunch of plyometrics to try and force some more strength and power, we regressed to intrinsic foot strengthening, 360-degree ankle work, and boring old calf raises. He worked his ass off for a year. He now describes the change in his running as, "I can actually feel my foot hitting the ground now. My whole leg from my butt to my foot feels like one unit moving behind me. It's like an entirely new leg."

This is the kind of work personal trainers should do better than anyone. Doctors would have wondered if he needed a brace, surgery, or told him to stop running entirely. Physical therapists wouldn't have had enough time with him to complete the work. The internet would have given him running drills. He needed a personal trainer. He told me he thought when we started training, we would just do a bunch of stations for cardio workouts, because that's what he had always done with trainers. I laughed. We are so much more capable than just putting seven stations of random exercises together. I'm dying for personal training to get away from this model of randomness, and that's what I'm hoping this book will teach to new trainers.

This is why the Comp Two is so critical. You don't need to get fancy. You don't need to know intricate stuff. You just need a strong grasp of the basics and know what you're looking for. If you have that, you'll be able to put fresh eyes on what your client might have been dealing with for ages. You will be able to see a new path for them to try, and it will always start with cleaning up the basics.

At the end of your Comp Two, you and your client should both have more information about their movement and fitness situation. Your client should feel like:

- They learned something about their body that they didn't know (or learned a new way to work on something they did already know).

• They had a more difficult and more focused workout than they can do themselves.

• The work was more enjoyable than working alone, even though the work itself was more difficult.

• They accomplished something they didn't know they could do.

• You saw their body as it is, were able to adjust to their body as it is, and saw a doable plan for the future. (They might not recognize this as anything other than feeling like their body isn't as ugly and monstrous as they imagined.)

• You gave them hope for improvement. This is the big one. People are always scared that we're gonna tell them they are a lost cause. If you show them concrete ways that they are already strong, and concrete ways that they could be stronger, they will leave feeling amazing. And someone who feels amazing will want to train with you again.

This goes without saying, but all of the above needs to be genuine. You're not just there to sugarcoat and sweet-talk vulnerable people into giving you their money. This is called scamming and although there are trainers and gyms who do this, you don't want to be one of them. One of the first trainers I ever worked alongside was a disgusting man. He would lie to his clients about their body fat percentage (telling them it was higher than it was) and tell them that they would never be able to do anything by themselves. He told them they *needed* to only train with him, because if they worked out alone they would fail. He BRAGGED TO ME about doing this. What a disgrace. (Incidentally, he also referred to me as "that bitch" when talking to our managers about me. Better proof than a DNA test that I really am 100% that bitch.)

Here's what I want to know about my client by the end of the Comp Two:

- Their strongest motor patterns and their weakest motor patterns.

- The way they like to be coached. Pay attention to their body language throughout. What makes them light up and try again? What makes them wince?

- Did their injuries show up the way the client described them in the Comp One? Maybe they weren't an issue like the client thought, or maybe they showed up differently than the client thought.

- In general, I want to feel like the two of us can get some great work done. If there's some reason I don't feel like I can promise that, I'll address it here. (Maybe they won't commit to a regular schedule, or maybe I got the sense that my coaching style isn't what they're looking for.)

I always wrap up a new client's first workout with a review. Here's what I thought was great and here's what I thought needed work. Here's where I intend to start your program, and here's what we probably don't need to focus on for now. Here's what I'd like you to start doing on your own, and here's what I'd rather you wait on until you're with me. I review every single exercise we worked on that day, explain why I flagged the things I did, and why I think other things are better than the client thought. Leave time to answer all their questions, and find out if they are interested in doing a few more sessions together.

If they are interested, try to schedule them pronto. The best time to get people on board with you is immediately after a fantastic workout, because they'll be experiencing that workout happiness in that moment. If they say they're unsure, I might see if they want to schedule just one more session with me. This is so we can create a workout together that specifically focuses on the weak points we just identified. Lots of people will jump on this, because buying one session is super low commitment. And if they still aren't sure? Say "No problem! I'm always around," and let them go.

From a sales perspective, you never want to let a potential client leave because they're immediately less likely to come back. People (businessmen) used to counsel me about this all the time. Always Be Closing, Sell Sell Sell, etc. But from a human perspective, a salesperson who won't let you leave is really fucking annoying. Let people leave. Lots of them will come back to you down the line.

That's an important part of being a trainer. It's a delayed gratification field. You will do two free sessions with someone and then they might not come back for a year. But after that? Permanent client. There are tons of reasons why someone might not immediately buy from you, and those reasons can always change. So don't be pissy if someone says no. If you did your job right, they got some great information from you in those two free sessions, and they'll remember that when it's time to look for more. Be patient and don't be a greedy asshole.

As a final note, you can use an abbreviated form of this assessment when you're teaching group ex classes. I always use the warm-up time to spy on people, especially anyone new in the class. Incorporate squats, lunges, pushes, pulls, and/or balance into your warm-up. Look quickly for ease of movement, control, whether they look confused or confident, speed and endurance, etc. Are they finishing the warm-up lunges alongside the more experienced people in class or are they falling behind? You'll develop an excellent eye for identifying everyone's level quite quickly, which will allow you to adapt your class plan on the fly.

So you've become a trainer, picked up clients, taken them through their first workout, and sold them a few sessions. What happens next? You need to keep them around. Let's talk about providing care and building trust with your new client.

TL;DR

1) A client's free workout is your best chance to show your skills in sixty minutes. Pay attention to them, learn to think fast, and don't get distracted. Remember, mobility, strength, and speed, in that order.

2) You don't have to demonstrate every exercise on Earth or do three sets of everything during their workout. It's too much work and too much information. And besides, you're not trying to fry them on day one.

3) Try to identify two or three things during the session that you could help them improve. Don't point out every single mistake they're making. Similarly, don't tell them everything is wonderful just to try and get in their good graces. Not only can people see through this, but they might also decide that if they're already so excellent, what do they need you for?

4) Give them a good challenge—people should realize that you offer something they haven't been able to do for themselves. But don't make everything too hard for them. There's a fine line between feeling challenged and feeling demoralized. One will train with you again. The other will not.

5) Ask other experienced trainers about their assessments and evaluations. Everyone trains a little bit differently, and this will help you figure out your own best way of assessing clients.

6) Make sure your client feels sensational at the end. Do not finish the session until they feel genuinely great.

Chapter Seven: Building Trust

Personal training, like all one-on-one service relationships, is built on trust. This is how you get clients and this is how you keep clients. Think of some times when you've been a patron, and how important trust was in those situations. For example, you trust that your massage therapist is never going to do anything to your naked body but massage it. You trust that your servers and bartenders are not going to spit into your food at your favorite restaurant. If anything unsavory happened in either of those situations, you'd be out at light speed and never return. In personal training, you trust that your trainer isn't going to hurt your body. The way you take care of people's most precious asset—their body—is the number one way they will develop and retain trust in you, so let's start there.

Doing no harm is an oath for doctors but it should be for trainers too. One of the most common things that people say to me when we meet is that they don't want to get hurt. Well, duh! No one wants to get hurt. We're always trying to avoid that. But many people have one distinct image of what personal trainers do, and that's hurt people. I had one person say that they aren't looking for a militant drill sergeant who screams at them and makes them do insane shit until they sob and wretch on the floor while peeing uncontrollably. I'm not sure how they heard about my sex life but I reassured them that I don't lead my professional life that way.

You'll do your best to prevent it, but injuries will happen if you're a trainer for long enough. I've given out plenty of small ones and a few biggies over the years. A torn calf muscle, an ACL tear, a dislocated shoulder, a concussion that I swear wasn't my fault. Lots of grumpy lower backs and tendonopathies. Even though that's about one major injury per six thousand sessions, which is pretty good, they still haunt me. But I reassure myself by knowing that sometimes shit happens in athletics, and that's ok. You can't promise someone that they won't ever get hurt with you. You just do the best you can to create a safe environment and that's it. If you operate in such a way that when someone gets hurt, you can look back and know that you used an appropriate exercise with proper warm-up and coaching, then you've done your job. When you're always creating thoughtful workouts and interactions with your clients, they'll understand those very rare times when things go wrong.

Preventing physical injury is part of the client-protection battle, but preventing emotional injury is another, and you have more control here. Body shaming is easier to do than you might think. First off, don't publicly body shame them, like talking about how doing this cardio is gonna help them lose weight, or don't they want to fit into their dress for the wedding? (I did this to a woman once. I was a brand new trainer and I said, when she stopped her set early, "Come on! Doing it to look amazing at the wedding!" She dropped her weight, turned to face me dead-on and said sternly, "That won't work on me. Don't do that." After all the blood returned to my body, I agreed, and haven't done it to anyone since.)

Shaming isn't just about fat and thin. We have all kinds of shitty, deeply ingrained biases towards people's bodies. Trust me, you do. Maybe you think older people are fragile, that women shouldn't lift big weights, or that kids shouldn't lift weights at all. A trainer once told a dear friend of mine that she just didn't think my friend's body would ever be able to learn a pushup. What the fuck? I've often heard trainers answer technique questions by saying, "Well when I do this, I do it this really hard way, but when YOU do it, you'll do it this much easier way." To me, that instantly reads as "You'll never be able to do what I can do," which, to me, is a form of body shaming. I always assume that my clients are on the way to becoming the strongest person on

Earth and I train them accordingly. Even things as minute as small workout tics can be embarrassing if you call them out. I once teased a woman about how she held her arms up like a bunny rabbit when doing squats and she was mortified. I still feel badly about it. No matter what, your clients need to be certain that you are not judging them—even about tiny things—and that you're on their side. The last thing you want is a trainer—someone who is supposed to bolster your self-image and self-efficacy—making you feel awful about yourself. If you don't truly believe in your clients, they'll know it. This is the primary way of building your client's trust in you.

Beyond keeping their body as safe as you can, you can earn your clients' trust in four other ways. If you want to slay your career, you need to cultivate and maintain all four kinds, at all times, with all your clients.

1. **Get to know them as a person.**
2. **Show up every time.**
3. **Give them great workouts.**
4. **Get other people to talk about you.**

The first is outlined in most of the book to this point. You talk to clients, learn about them as a human, show genuine interest in their lives, and don't treat them like a wallet. They're coming to you with a problem, and you're trying to determine whether you could help solve that problem. A great conversation goes a long way towards demonstrating that you might be the solution they need. And to be clear, just being chatty, or talking about yourself the whole time, is not the same thing as a great conversation. Ask pointed questions and remember the answers. Because the next time you see them, if you know which foot was the one they broke in 1997, and remember to ask how their daughter's dance recital went over the weekend, you'll go a long way to proving your desire to know and help *them*, and *specifically* them. That's the personal part of personal training.

Although I hope this would be self-evident to the industry, it's not. The national personal training chains are not personal at all. So if you're considering starting your career with one of them, you should know that it works more like this: The trainers don't assess the clients themselves. They're handed a group of clients, every half hour or hour, and a series of workouts for the week. Every one of the company's thousands of customers does those workouts that week. Then everyone repeats the process the following week.

Yes, if you take a job at one of these places, you'll have more work right away, unlike the scenarios I described in the beginning of this book. But I want to be so clear: it's not personal training. Even if it's one trainer with one client who is following the national corporate protocol, this isn't personal training. This is a giant group exercise class. The trainer isn't deciding on the fitness needs for one person. They're reading generic exercises off of a screen and assigning them to one person. Big difference. And, by the way, the stories I've heard about the big chains teaching their trainers a specific sales protocol to make women cry, in order to sell them a larger pack of training sessions? Fuck me. I hate that so much. Be extremely cautious before accepting a job at these places. They suck.

Because of this trash, people are often surprised by what personal training is like at our gym, and other great gyms who operate like we do. We always emphasize that personal training is, in fact, supposed to be personal! It is supposed to look at one person in great detail, identify their individual movement patterns and habits, and create a program that addresses their particular strengths and weaknesses. That program and plan should change regularly as you learn more about your client, as they improve, and as their goals change.

I'm just gonna keep saying it: **personal training is supposed to be personal.** So the first way to earn your client's trust is to get to know them and their bodies specifically.

The second way to earn your clients' trust is self-explanatory. Show up. Every. Time. Don't skip out when you don't feel like it. Don't move session times for your own convenience. Don't late cancel people. How To Lose A Client In Ten Days? Give them the slightest doubt about whether you'll show up for your next session. Give them one reason to think that their business isn't important to you. Like the mistake you banged in college, they'll be gone by sunrise.

This whole book so far has been about knowing the client as a person, but now we're gonna talk about knowing the client as a body. The third way you earn trust as a personal trainer is the exercise. The workouts have to be good, every time. You have to know what you're talking about and communicate that to the client, every time. They should always know what the plan is. A great understanding of the human body and how it moves is critical to being an excellent trainer.

You need to understand anatomy and biomechanics in order to be an effective and safe trainer, so I've created a study guide for you. This list is what I would consider a comprehensive and sound base of knowledge for a trainer to bring to a client. To be clear, this goes way beyond what the certification tests require. You need to learn them anyway. I consider these basic and standard.

We're starting with joints from the bottom, because you cannot understand how a body moves unless you look at the feet first.

- **Feet and ankles:** Understand the three arches of the foot, the way the foot is supposed to spread out on the floor to bear weight, and the natural pronation/supination that occurs with gait. Understand ankle dorsiflexion, plantarflexion, inversion, eversion, and the Achilles tendon. Also understand that foot and ankle function has an enormous effect on all of the joints above it, particularly knees, hips, pelvis, and spine. Limited big toe dorsiflexion is a big problem. Keep an eye out for it.

• **Knees:** Understand the patellar and quad tendons, the large ligaments (ACL, MCL, PCL, LCL), and the way the femur and tibia connect with each other throughout knee flexion and extension. Understand tibial rotation. Recognize the knees as the stabilizing joints for the ankles and hips and understand how that affects the forces traveling through them.

• **Hips:** Understand the myriad planes of motion of the hip—flexion, extension, internal/external rotation, abduction, adduction, and understand how these planes directly impact the pelvis and spine. A strong knowledge of the three glute muscles, especially maximus and medius. Particular knowledge of hip extension and internal rotation is critical in a population that sits all the time and rarely runs at high speed. (In other words, nearly everyone.)

• **Pelvis:** Recognize the way that pelvic movement is meant to be independent of hip and spine movement. Understand anterior and posterior pelvic tilts and why they develop. (Tilts are not the big deal everyone makes of them! Your pelvis is supposed to tilt. The only issue is if the person *can't* get out of one orientation or the other.)

• **Spine and neck:** Understand flexion, extension, and rotation of each part of the spine and neck. See the spine as an incredibly strong and resilient part of the body, not a fragile bomb waiting to go off. Recognize the way that poor foot push-off, poor hip extension, and poor foot/hip strength in general can cause serious spinal dysfunction and pain.

• **Shoulders:** Understand the planes of motion—flexion, extension, internal/external rotation, abduction, and adduction. Study deeply the rotator cuff muscles and their function. (Great knowledge of the rotator cuff will serve you extremely well as a trainer.) Have a good concept of scapular movement and how it impacts the neck, shoulders, elbows, and wrists.

• **Elbows:** Understand flexion, extension, and rotation at the joint. Similar to the knee, understand that the elbow is the stabilizing link between the mobile shoulder and wrist. Recognize that common elbow dysfunction (tennis/golfer's elbow) is generally a symptom of poor wrist/forearm strength combined with poor scapular stability/strength.

• **Wrists and hands:** Understand flexion, extension, rotation, abduction, adduction, plus thumb abduction and adduction. Understand how grip affects the elbow, shoulder, scapula, and spine.

So that's basic joint movement. Now, the muscle groups you have to know and understand. Again, from the bottom up.

• **Intrinsic foot muscles.** The base of all strong movement everywhere in the body.

• **Calves and shins: gastrocnemius, soleus, anterior and posterior tibialis.** Weak calves lead to knee, hip, and back problems in walkers and especially runners. Anterior and posterior tib greatly affect foot mechanics.

• **Quads.** Understanding the pros and cons of their dominance.

• **Hamstrings.** Become obsessed with the hamstrings in anyone who sits all the time.

• **Hip adductors.** Everyone forgets about these. They are a critical component of hip and spine health.

• **Hip abductors**. One of the keystones of core strength.

• **Gluteus Maximus.** Become obsessed with glute max in everyone, particularly in extension.

• **The Core.** Recognize that this includes all of the abdominal muscle groups, the pelvic floor, the deep spinal muscles, the diaphragm, and the hip muscles.

• **Lats and Traps.** Many trainers have a weak understanding of how these two muscles have a massive impact on shoulder health.

• **Scapular stabilizers besides the traps.** Everyone forgets about these too; serratus, rhomboids, levators.

• **The Rotator Cuff.** Again, an excellent understanding of the rotator cuff will be one of the most valuable assets to you as a trainer.

• **Deltoids, Biceps, Triceps**. Just because they're vanity muscles doesn't mean they're not critical function muscles as well!

- **Forearms.** The arms can only be as strong as the weakest link in the chain. A weak grip automatically limits upper body strength.

- **The brain.** The most important muscle. Study some basic neurology, especially pain science, motivation, and the psychology of self-esteem.

You do not have to be an expert in all of the above. But you do need to understand each of these structures and their function, because absolutely nothing in the human body is an independent organism. The best way I can put it is that everything working properly depends on everything else working properly. This is the most important concept to understand about the human body.

Here's an example of why: When I was a new, inexperienced trainer, I thought it was stupid to do isolated movements like clamshells or glute bridges. I would confidently say, "Listen, nothing in the body works by itself. Those clamshells aren't going to fix your barbell squats. If you want to fix your barbell squats then you need to barbell squat."

I was half right: nothing in the body works by itself. But I was half dead wrong, too. Each individual part of the body MUST be able to function well by itself before it can function well in the group. Let's say you have a client who never feels a glute bridge in their glutes; only in their quads or lower back. That means their glutes are firing weakly and/or with poor timing. If that person barbell squats, their glutes will not provide maximum effort in the lift. They will be hyper-dependent on the quads and lower back. This is a great way for your client to get hurt while squatting.

The way to regenerate that lost glute power is to go back and isolate the glutes until they're firing with strength at the initiation of movement. As the foundation of the lift is correct, the quality of lift will skyrocket.

The body is a phenomenal compensator, which I used to think was a great thing. It can be a great thing, but it also hides the problems that cause the problems. We talked about this in the last chapter as well, with the man who could squat 700 pounds on his back, but not do a partial-range, single-leg, bodyweight squat. He needed more isolated work in order to build up the whole work.

Studying the whole and being able to break it down into parts to identify the weak links is the definition of personal training. The glute max MUST be able to extend independently, without extra help from the hamstrings or lower back. The calves MUST be able to push someone into plantarflexion without the quads kicking in and the knees buckling. The scapulae MUST be able to depress and retract, without the upper traps doing the most instead. Each muscle and joint is supposed to contribute a certain percentage of movement. When one muscle or joint is weak, and another muscle or joint is constantly being asked to over-contribute, everyone is gonna have a bad time. (Helloooooo, tendinopathy, strains, spasms, and pain) When each part of the chain proves that it can work independently, then you know it will contribute to the movement as a whole.

Providing good, thoughtful workouts is a major trust-builder. When you can understand movement patterns and how they impact each other, you'll be able to evaluate new clients in a breeze. When you can confidently say, "That looks weaker in the left hip, is that how it feels to you?" they'll agree, and wonder how you just did a magic trick. It's not magic, it's that you're educated and paying attention to them. This is one reason that good personal training is expensive: a knowledgeable trainer is invaluable in identifying someone's individual movement patterns and problems. I can see poor hip extension, weak feet, or scapular instability from a mile away. This is why it breaks my heart when someone tells me they're not gonna train with me, they're gonna go to one of those clown-ass chain gyms because they're cheaper.

Yes, I'm expensive, but I know that my decades of education and time invested in the field are going to be well-worth it to my clients. Every time someone tells me they're going to go to a national chain for cheap training, an angel loses its wings and also ends up with back pain.

The final spoke of the trust-building wheel is other people. You can have other people create trust for you. How? By regularly introducing your clients and class attendees to each other and to the wider gym community, even people who aren't your clients. When other people tell your client that they think you're great, your client will feel proud that they get to work with you. It's like if someone loves the same movie you do, you discuss it thoroughly and come out confirming that it really is a great movie.

The best is when the people start lovingly trash-talking you. That's when you know you've made it. They'll bond over the exercises they hate, your cheerful demeanor while assigning deadly things, and whether your class playlists really need to contain so much of Britney Spears's catalog. As hilarious as it is, letting people relentlessly shit-talk you is the surest road to success. A person who hears about you from a friend they trust is going to automatically trust you more. If they hear about you from an entire group in the locker room after you give a great class? They'll be your client by tomorrow.

The dream personal training pipeline is to meet someone, start to see who they are personality-wise in the Comp One, start to see who they are body-wise in the Comp Two, and then take that knowledge into a few sessions that blow their minds. Most personal trainers convert one or two out of ten people into regular clients. But when someone likes spending time with you, gets a workout that's tailored to some of their issues, demonstrates an improvement in those issues, leaves feeling like they worked on exactly what they need help with, and trusts your ideas, they will sign up immediately, no matter what you cost. When

I switched my evaluation style for the Comp One, and got better at running Comp Twos, my conversion rate went from 10% to 90% over the course of about a year, even at one of the most expensive gyms in Boston.

So someone bought a whole pack of sessions with you and they're on board for the ride. Congrats! You've gotten a new client! Now, you gotta keep them around. This happens with great workouts and great company. Let's talk about nurturing client relationships.

TL;DR

1) To make real sales, believe in the fantastic service that you're offering. This is different from believing in the product you're selling. The first is about them. The second is about you. Make it about them.

2) People will trust you when you see them for who they are. Learn how to read people fast. This comes by asking them thoughtful questions and actually being interested in—and listening to—the responses.

3) Try to solve someone's problem right away. Don't make them buy personal training before trying to solve their problem. See if you can help them in the very first appointment. And if you're not the solution, tell them that and point them to the person who is.

4) Don't assume they trust you simply because you're the trainer. It doesn't work that way. They're almost always inclined to DIStrust you for the same reason. You need to prove yourself. Learn your shit.

Chapter Eight: Nurturing Client Relationships

Personal training is an unusual field in many ways, but the trainer/client relationship is one of the most unusual parts. My friends who work outside of the gym are always astonished by my stories. They're like, "You're going to your client's house for dinner? You're traveling with them to see the Celtics in Florida? They loaned you their penthouse in London?" Yes, yes, and yes.

You will develop wonderful relationships with your clients—deep, caring, personal, relationships. It's one of the best parts of the job for me. I spend every work day hanging out with my friends the whole time. Every hour a new friend comes in! Training is more social than massage and esthetics, and you see people way more often than a hairdresser, so it's uniquely positioned for you and your clients to live your lives together. I see most of my clients more often than their families do. And during rest periods in our workouts, we talk about most everything.

As I have said a hundred times (but will keep saying), you have to have a friendly relationship with your clients. You have to listen to them and care about their outcomes if you're going to have a long relationship together. Knowing more about a client's life helps you make better decisions about how to train them. What kind of person are they? Are they a 5am rise 'n' grind or a "Don't even offer me a session before 10am" retiree? Are they a family person who cooks dinner every night? Or do they have a difficult home life? What do they do for hobbies? What are their priorities? The workouts need to fit the personalities.

A rise 'n' grind type is not likely to enjoy casual, laidback workouts. He will like data, programs, information, stuff he can enter into his Apple watch tracking app. Someone who craves peace and serenity in their body does not want to do a metcon ever. And it's not just personality either. Knowing their life outside the gym matters. For example, my clients who have a difficult home life are liable to come in somewhere between stressed and panicked on any given day. Panicked days are not the days to attempt deadlift PRs or anaerobic threshold workouts. You'll blow every circuit in your client's body.

Paying attention to details will give you some insight into how someone would like to train. This is true in the macro sense (what kind of workouts they might enjoy the most in general) and in the micro sense (how will any given part of their life affect them during that day's workout). You are training the WHOLE person, not just the physical meat and bones inside them. You need to understand how they like to be spoken to and what their triggers are. Knowing the person's training style and lifestyle allows you to tailor each workout to what they need that day. You can program your client's sessions ahead of time all you want, but you'll never be able to predict when someone will come in after being in a car accident, when they just got served divorce papers, or have suffered a horrible and very public humiliation. (All things which have happened in my career.)

I often joke that this job is 50% exercise, 30% friendship, and 20% psychotherapy. If your clients don't want to hang out with you, they aren't likely to train with you either. You will absolutely act as a therapist, so your emotional intelligence needs to be off the charts. But you're there to exercise of course. So you need to understand when to stop chatting and work, when to stop working and chat, when to back up your client when they're struggling, and when to push back against them as needed.

A big part of nurturing great relationships with your clients is being able to listen without offering advice, not talking about yourself all the time, being non-judgmental about what they share with you, and then—this is huge—not sharing that information with other people. ESPECIALLY spouses/family members. If I train spouses in separate sessions, I never disclose to one spouse what the other spouse told me unless it's something simple like weekend plans or a dinner reservation. Same with a parent/child. You never know what is secret between them—or what is supposed to be a secret from you—so treat everything like a secret. (Yes, I learned this the hard way, multiple times.)

What on earth could be so secret that would come up during a workout with a personal trainer? Let's see. Marriage bickering, rebellious teenagers at home, the challenges of having a new baby, mental health struggles, money difficulties, sick parents, estranged siblings, illegal things happening at work, etc. All the normal stuff.

But you'll also hear plenty of stuff that will make your eyebrows want to shoot through your skull. I've had alcoholic clients and drug-addicted clients, or those telling me about their drug-addicted family members. I've had clients confess to affairs, confide that they're in an unsafe domestic situation, or tell me that they are closeted gay and hidden by a straight marriage. I am usually the first to know when someone is pregnant, when someone is considering divorce, when someone has lost their job, or is making a massive career move. I've had several female clients stuck in bad marriages because their husband has all the money. I know how much money my clients make, how much their houses are worth, and what they intend to leave to their kids. People will share health scares, cancer diagnoses, dementia diagnoses, and all kinds of concerns about their spouses, siblings, and children. I told you before that your clients will see you more than they see their own families; twice I've had to secretly locate a client's family members to share that my client was showing clear signs of dementia. With their kids living across the country, it might be months or even years before they see it.

Exercise is rarely serious, but the exercise relationship is super serious. If you're in this field for long enough, you will be asked to provide a space for some really intense shit. As I said, I try my hardest not to offer advice, definitely try not to offer my opinion, and simply to be available to hold whatever they're asking me to hold. I do generally feel free to ask questions about whatever people have already chosen to share. Remember, people look forward to training with you. It's a luxury. They *want* to talk with you about their lives, since you're not usually otherwise involved in it. You're a safe space for them. So don't be shy! In between rounds of deadlifts, ball slams, and Turkish get-ups, you have a surprising amount of time to ask questions and chat about the answers.

I do recommend digging deep from time to time. (Be aware of who's around if you are asking personal or sensitive questions, because someone will always be eavesdropping on your session.) I always use a preface statement first when I have a more personal question. Something like, "Definitely don't share all the details, but..." or "By all means tell me to fuck off if you don't want to talk about this..." or something similar. Because even if they brought it up, they might not want to have this conversation on the floor. So you want to give them an easy out. If they indicate that they don't want to answer, immediately say, "No problem!" and be ready with their next instruction.

Debates might arise, as they often do with sensitive topics. Use your discretion in moving a session along if it's getting caught up in something heated. And for heaven's sake, don't argue with your clients on the floor. If I have a client sharing different political views from mine, I'll always say, "Oh, ok!" or ask them a follow-up question about their thoughts. I'd never start a debate or share my opposing views. It's not what I'm there for. That being said, if someone says something racist, phobic, sexist, etc, don't be afraid to call it out. I've definitely intercepted some racist remarks in the past. My partner Eric used to train a powerful man who would ask Eric how badly he wanted to sleep with each of his female employees (or if he already had). This man would leer after their bodies and ask Eric for his opinion on what sex with each of them might be like. Fuck that. Eric got out of there as soon as he could. Just because a client is paying for your time doesn't mean they're entitled to say whatever garbage they want and force you to agree with it.

It's not to say that every session is full of moaning and depression and misogyny. Far from it! My clients and I are laughing for 90% of their time. But because you see people so often, you'll be acutely aware of their day-to-day lives, and that means they'll occasionally be coming in for workouts while really going through it at home. You'll have sessions while the person is grieving a recently deceased family member, or they just walk through the door sobbing and you have no idea why. It will put you in a weird place to offer support—in some ways you know more about them than most of their friends, and in other ways you don't totally feel like a friend because there's always a professional distance. They may or may not tell you what's going on, so you might just be sitting in the middle of the gym with a sobbing client. What do I do in those situations? I always ask the person what kind of workout they're looking for. Some high-intensity cardio to help burn out a few of those powerful emotions? A slow, delicate session, designed not to frazzle a single nerve? Or just take a walk together? This is why trainers need to always be able to pivot a session in an instant. I even had one woman say, "Honestly? I desperately need a drink." It was Christmas Eve and she was my last person, so we left the gym and had martinis during her hour. Ready for anything!

What **can't** you talk about on the floor with clients? Well, that depends on the trainer. I only have one real boundary, which is that you may not talk shit to me about someone else nearby. One nosy former client used to loudly say things like, "Do you think that girl on the stairmaster is anorexic?" or "Is that the woman whose daughter died last year?" I was not sad to stop training him. Another client used to say things like, "Wow, that woman is running even though she's fat!" or would compare another member's body to her own and ask me my opinion on who looked better. Hell. Fucking. No.

Some of my coworkers do have conversational boundaries. Eric won't talk about sex, politics, or money with his clients. I talk about all three of those things extremely regularly. I am more casual and friendly with my clients, whereas he tends to keep more distance. It's on you to decide what works for you. There are pros and cons to both, and different clients will like different approaches. Some of his clients wouldn't enjoy my chattiness, and some of my clients wouldn't enjoy Eric's distance. This doesn't mean that Eric doesn't do every single thing that I've listed here about how to promote great client relationships. He does. But he leaves it at the gym and I love building relationships outside of the gym. The bottom line is trust, however that gets cultivated.

You are always working to build and maintain trust with your clients. The trainer-client dynamic works best when you have complete faith in each other. You'll be able to tell right away when a client doesn't have faith in you. They're suspicious of what you're asking them to try, they tell you that all their trainers in the past have hurt them, they contradict your opinion by spouting something they read on the internet, they pooh-pooh your safety suggestions as if they were a personal challenge. All red flags. Pay attention to this. It's not a big issue at first. But if you can't get them to trust you and your training process after a few sessions, try talking with them about it. See if you can ease their mind about your work. If you can't, hand them off to another trainer. They might have a better connection with that person, which is better for everyone.

Trust is the secret to the personal relationship, but it's also the secret to the workout relationship. The more your client trusts you, the more freedom you'll have to guide them through difficult exercises. This includes things they might have had trouble with in the past, unusual skills they might be unfamiliar with, or movements that scare them but you know are critical to their success. This is especially important in the beginning, when clients are either afraid of getting hurt or afraid that you can't help them. If someone does have pain, even just sore muscles, they will react to it differently if they trust you than if they don't. That's why the 360-degree relationship development matters. Talk well with your clients so you can work well with your clients.

If it makes you uncomfortable to imagine diving deeply into someone's extramarital affair or personal finances when they're supposed to be exercising, don't worry. You can (and should) choose the distance you want to keep between you and your clients. The trust can be there no matter what distance you decide on. Like all relationships, trust is built in lots of ways, not just by talking about hard shit. Here are some easy things that will also nurture the relationship in a positive way but not require you to be a therapist:

- Showing up on time

- Being reliable with your schedule

- Always giving a good session

- Answering their communications promptly

- Keeping their private thoughts private

- Asking them thoughtful questions about themselves

- If you're videoing or photographing them for any reason (usually social media or gym promotion), always asking permission to film it and to use it, even if they've given you permission before

- Remembering their personal details

- Being non-judgmental

- Holding them accountable to their work in the gym

- Not shit-talking one client to another client. The client who's on the receiving end will start wondering if you talk about them with other people.

- When you are aggravated by one person, don't let it bleed into another person's session. When you are aggravated in general, don't let it bleed into all your sessions that day. (And boy can this be hard. We will go more into this in chapter twelve.) When people do infuriate you, do what we all do and send capital-letter rage texts to your best friend instead.

A quick note on the topic of being annoyed at work, because this is part of the trust diagram. It took me years to realize that when I complain to a client about being tired at work, or complain about how many sessions I have that day, or complain about having a difficult client at the end of the day—complaints I would make to any friend, and my clients are friends—it's a bad professional look. I can't believe it took me so long to recognize this, but it makes your client feel like shit. Of course it does! When you say you wish you could go home, you're literally telling them that you don't want to be there with them. That sucks.

I don't advocate lying, toxic positivity, or being a Yes Person for your clients. You can definitely be honest about your current state of being. But you always need to indicate that you are looking forward to their session and enjoy your time together while you're in it. I've caught myself saying, "UGH, this morning I would have done ANYTHING to not go in to work today." Meanwhile my client who's paying $135 for me to go in to work today is listening to me say I wish I were somewhere else. Sometimes they'll uncomfortably respond, "You could have cancelled me!" It's embarrassing, an awful way to treat customers, and a great way to lose customers. If they don't feel like you really want to be there with them, they won't remain your client for long. Some trainers get burned out to the point that all their sessions make them miserable. If that happens, faking it will only make things worse for everyone. If you get to that point, take a break, or make a change. Faking job enjoyment in a one-to-one service career is difficult and disingenuous.

There's one other way to build and maintain great relationships with your clients: outside communication. If they give me permission, I text with my clients the way I text with my outside friends. I'll send them pictures of stuff that reminds me of them, I'll check in on their sore knee over the weekend, I'll ask them to send me updates from the best parts of their vacations. I often have lunch or dinner with clients. Every January, I write a thank-you card to everyone who did at least one session with me the previous year. I summarize what I think were the most important things we worked on, congratulate them on doing hard work, and point out the things that have improved. I strongly recommend making this your own practice as well. People love to hear what you think has gone well for them. Moreover, they are keeping you employed. It's nice to say thank you.

All of this communication and friendshipping does come with some professional risks. Especially, I'm sorry to say, if you're a female trainer.

There's a world of gossip out there, because some people have very little to do. People have gossiped some appalling and completely untrue things about me, and several coworkers have experienced same. It seems to happen more to my female coworkers than my male ones. (Hmmmm.)

I've had some wives pissed that I cheerfully text their husbands (no matter how mundane the texts), and I've had some men mistake our professional friendship for more than that. A female trainer I know was once asked out by a client after a session. She said no, and then he followed her around on her errands for the rest of the day trying to get her to change her mind. That same woman also had a married male client start bringing her gold watches, jewelry, flowers, iPads. Eesh. Yes, people will give you holiday gifts or tips. It shouldn't be all the time, and it shouldn't be weird. You'll know if it's being given professionally or with another agenda.

More than one man has bought training sessions with me specifically to use that time to hit on me and/or ask me out. The first time it happened I was totally blindsided and trapped in an office when he sprung the invite on me. I instantly felt cheap and worthless. I'd been trying my hardest to plan his workouts and give him good training sessions, as I always try to do, only to find out he was just biding his time to try and nail me. Never cared about my fitness advice, couldn't give a shit about my work. I felt incredibly stupid.

Another man I'd been training for maybe six months asked me one day if I'd be willing to only wear skirts while we train together. After picking my jaw up off the floor, I told him no. He said, "Why not?" and I said, "Because I'm not your doll, and I'm not here to look cute for you." He wrote me an email later that night which began with, "Mia, it really hurt my feelings today when you said that you didn't want to be my doll."

He managed to get even creepier and I got out of the situation as soon as I could. I should have ended it long before I did, because I dreaded working with him. Ultimately I kept him on for too long because I really needed the work. As I said, that can happen in this field. But now I know that it's more important to feel safe at work than to get an extra $80 a week. If someone gives you the ick and you can't shake it, follow your gut and end the relationship. Hey, if you're wondering? This man was a Harvard Medical School gynecologist. This information is what the vomit emoji was made for.

Another guy, who was not my client for long, once had a session with me at six in the morning. He came in and I said, "Hey, Kevin! How are you this morning?" He replied, "I slept horribly. Last night I was having sex with my wife and all of a sudden you popped into my head because of our early session today. I couldn't get you out of my head and it ruined my sex and my night."

Sir, this is a Wendy's. I absolutely never needed to hear this story. In the least surprising twist of all time, he stopped training with me because—he said this out loud to me—he didn't like taking orders from a woman.

Another married man started texting me photos of him in his underwear, asking if I would give my "professional opinion" on his body progress. I told him to stop texting me and that I did not ever ask to receive naked photos from him. He said, feelings hurt, "I'm not naked. I'm in my underwear." Oh, that's fine then. This response is what the eye-roll emoji was made for.

There's one other aspect of trainer-client relationships, and it's an important one: Sex. Straight, gay, bi, fluid, it doesn't matter. If you work as a trainer for long enough, the option for sex is gonna enter the picture somewhere. I guarantee it. A client will develop a crush on you, or you'll develop a crush on a client. A gym member might be feeling you out, or a manager will shoot their shot. It's almost inevitable, and mostly it doesn't bother me personally. If a person interacts with enough other people, there's bound to be chemistry along the way. The problems come when someone decides to do something about it.

I have flirted with clients, gym members, coworkers, and bosses—but never slept or hooked up with any of them except one. (Should we have done it? Absolutely not. Then again, we've been together for sixteen years now, so I have no regrets.) But it happens all the time in the industry. The stories of trainers and clients regularly having sex make me cringe. Listen to me: Do not have sex with your clients!!! Do not have sex with your single clients!!! Do not have sex with your married clients!!! Do not have sex with your situationship clients!!! End the client part of it first. Then you can have sex with them all you want if you're both down. You fall in love with a gym member or client or coworker, well, that's awesome for both of you. It's a normal place to meet a partner. I fell in love with my boss. But sleeping with lots of clients or gym members just because you can? That will come back in a way you do not like. A gym I used to work at lost three trainers and two clients because of a complicated sexual pentagon and the gossip was *rampant*. Do not recommend.

Let me be clear: friendly communication, if it truly is harmless and intention-less, will rarely be interpreted incorrectly. But you'll need to be paying attention anyway. Part of a trainer's EQ is knowing that you're always staying within the boundaries of any given client or work relationship. You will need to keep an eagle eye for signs that you've crossed a boundary with a client. I had one man pissed at me for sending him a text at 11pm. He didn't want to explain to his wife that his trainer was sending him late-night texts. (It was a text about scheduling, but that didn't matter. I heard him loud and clear.)

My clients also know that I love to wear wacky outfits for concerts and events. So I had another male client ask me for a picture when I was going to the Britney Spears concert, which I happily sent. He was horrified by my skimpy outfit and the fact that I was standing, non-sexually, on a bed for the photo and lit into me about it. He had literally asked for a picture, so I didn't think I had done anything wrong. But without any context for our relationship, all that looks like is your personal trainer sending you slutty pictures at night. (Those are my words, not his. He was lovely about it, even though he was super mad.) This actually happened with another client as well, when he asked about my outfit for the Lady Gaga concert. So much for learning my lesson!

Personal training is a "hot" field. In other words, it's a lot of hot people working with hot clients who share interests and get sweaty and spend a lottttt of time together. It's not unusual for things to go wrong, as some of my stories above will indicate. If you're the kind of person (like me) who loves to shit-talk, flirt, sass, and generally be boisterous, you'll need to be extra careful. Check in with people if a joke lands badly or if your words don't come out the right way. There's never a wrong time for a "I'm sorry, I didn't intend to say that that way." You never want to leave any doubt as to your intentions. And if your intentions weren't great and you know it, you better be like DNA and check yourself before you wreck yourself. Remember that your reputation as a trainer is the most valuable thing you have and if you lose it, it is awfully hard to get it back without starting over in a new place.

And what about sexual harassment, sexual advances, aggressive text messages, etc, from your clients? I mean, it's a bad scene. You do not and should not have to put up with anything that makes you uncomfortable or feel unsafe. I dumped the guy who wanted me to wear skirts, the guy who sent me naked pics, the guy who trained with me just to ask me out, and I have reported two managers and one coworker for sexual harassment over the years. Never tolerate abusive behavior being directed at you. It does not matter if you've flirted back with your client or not. Do not let them treat you like a piece of meat for them to come visit when they feel like it.

Professional relationships that are also friendly will have gray areas. This is always true. For me, getting to experience deep, beautiful, consensual friendships with so many people I adore is well-worth the accidental missteps I've had on the way. I still have lunches and dinners with clients one-on-one, but I'm more careful of the optics than I used to be. My client-relationship boundary is that if I'm hanging out with a client, then anyone on earth—my partner, their spouse, other gym employees, someone's kids, etc—could suddenly show up, see what we were doing, and not have any questions about it. If someone would wonder what we were doing there, we shouldn't be there. You'll have your own ways of establishing boundaries, and whatever boundaries you set are gonna be the right ones. I will caution here that the closer you get with your clients, the blurrier the professional/friendly lines become and you will need to be prepared for that. We will talk about this more when we go over handling difficult client situations.

The client relationship is one of my favorite parts of being a personal trainer. My clients are my dear friends, and it is a dream to feel like my work is making a difference to my friends. Literally making my friends' lives better. But remember—and this is the key to the whole thing—you are doing a job first. In the gym setting, you're not exactly equal. You're a service provider to the person who needs the service. It means that the session is about them, in all ways. This can be weird when you're dying to just launch into conversation with one of your besties, but resist. They're there to do work, and so are you. When you're off the clock, on equal friendship footing again, and not asking them to do asymmetrically-weighted Bulgarian split squats where they hate you for ten minutes straight, *that's* when you can dive back in. Maintain this distancing triangle: treating the client as an important client in the session, as an important friend out of the session, and never as a sexual partner, and you'll always finish on top.

Metaphorically-speaking, that is.

TL; DR

1) Your clients are your most important work asset. Building and nurturing your relationships with them is a critical—and super fun!—part of the work. Invest time in it outside the gym.

2) You decide your boundaries and then stick to them. Some trainers, like me, are perfectly happy to socialize outside the gym with clients. Others do not. But if you do, be aware of the scene you're presenting publicly. Don't let people start wondering what you're up to.

3) Do not have sex with your clients. If there is a mutual, consensual, sexual relationship building, end the client part of it first.

4) Being fully engaged in the client relationship does not allow them to hit on you, harass you, or say any kind of phobic or tasteless comment to you. You aren't a puppet, punching bag, or object for them. Don't be afraid to stand up for yourself or ask for help from a supervisor if you need it.

5) Remember that during a session, the friendship part of things shifts a bit. You're not there to gab or talk about yourself. Save that for after the session, or for socializing outside the gym.

6) Enjoy the social aspect of your job! It's a privilege to be able to meet and interact with people from so many walks of life. You'll learn so much from your clients and they will remain your clients if they love their time with you as well.

Chapter Nine: The Business Side of Training

Money will always be on your mind as a trainer, because the financial side of personal training is strange. In a normal job, you agree in advance to a set salary and benefits, paid by your company. You get paid time off, personal time, regular raises, and performance/end-of-year bonuses. It's all part of the gig from the start.

In personal training, you agree to a salary of *shrug*, with a host of benefits ranging from *no one knows* to *depends on how long you can sustain earning below minimum wage*. There's no such thing as a raise or annual performance bonus. You might get paid time off in a couple years, but you have to earn it to get it and you have to keep earning it to retain it. If you want to work less, or take vacations, please set fire to the whole idea of paid benefits. And while your sessions are technically paid out by your company, there's no getting around the fact that the people actually paying your salary are your clients. If your client forgets to buy a new bundle of sessions, you don't get paid. If they late-cancel and refuse to take responsibility for it, you don't get paid. If they go on vacation, you don't get paid. When a three-time-a-week client stops training with you, that's an $8,000 annual salary cut, just like that.

All of which means that being able to talk money with your clients is absolutely vital. It's not always comfortable, but it is vital. You need to be able to ask them to pay for new training packages and pay for late cancellations. They need to understand that if they're constantly changing their schedule last minute, it affects your ability to book other people, which affects both your salary and your benefits. That's a conversation I've had to have many times, and people can get mad. Training is expensive, and some people feel that their money is more important than yours. You have to stand up for yourself. This is another great reason to cultivate and maintain excellent relationships with your clients. People are much less likely to be mad about pay when you have a friendly, thoughtful relationship with each other.

Besides the one-on-one client money problems, there are some affiliate money challenges which come part and parcel with being a personal trainer, especially if you work for a gym instead of for yourself. A few of the uncomfortable business situations you'll find yourself in include:

- Your gym's cancellation policies

- Whether difficult clients are worth the cash

- The clients you love but have a money dispute with

- Being accommodating with clients but not letting them walk all over you just because they're paying you

- Separating yourself from a shit gym manager or corporate office that your clients don't like

- Being a popular trainer at a gym with unpopular policies

- People who want your time and expertise for free

- Staying within the limits of your job and qualifications and not overstepping into other fields

- The opposite of the previous one, which is holding your ground when other fields step into YOUR area of expertise with bad/old information (this is usually doctors, but can also be massage therapists, acupuncturists, chiropractors, etc who do not have fitness training).

In my career, I have screwed up every single bullet point above, so I've got advice for all of it. But the main point is, there's no avoiding the money part of the job. Even when you have a good boss who will help you handle money stuff that gets out of control (and a good boss is not always guaranteed), you're going to have to do plenty of negotiation yourself.

Let's start with cancellations. There's a standard rule in personal training (and most 1-1 service fields) of a twenty-four hour cancellation policy. If someone cancels late, they get charged full price for the session. It's harsh, but essential. I hate charging people to not get a workout. It makes me feel shitty. And at the same time, every time I don't charge a session, I earn less money, the gym earns less money, and it puts my benefits at risk.

Health and PTO benefits as a trainer are tied to hitting a certain number of sessions per quarter. At many gyms, you need to average thirty-five hours a week in order to begin receiving—and continue to receive—health benefits. And this doesn't mean spending thirty-five hours a week at the gym. That would be lovely. No, it means thirty-five hours of paid PT sessions. Typically, having thirty-five to forty sessions in a week means that I am at the gym for at least fifty hours a week. And this thirty-five hour requirement is written in stone. Gym management does not play around when it comes to benefits. If you don't hit your numbers, your benefits are immediately rescinded until the next review.

At my old gym, I saw coworkers come in at a 34.95-hour quarterly average and that was it. There was no recovery. It's a long three months to get benefits back again. Corporate honey badger don't give a shit. For this reason alone, cancellations can be brutal. Keeping every single session that you have booked is essential, especially since the quarterly review will include the naturally slower times like summer and the end-of-year holidays. During those times, you know that you're starting in a deficit, and every cancellation makes the deficit worse. We had five full-time trainers at my old gym, and all of us were constantly worried about our hours in spite of having lots of clients. When benefits can be taken away any time, you never feel comfortable. This is one reason I always say that if you want to travel a ton, personal training is not the career for you.

Cancellations can also be awkward. It's tough to say, "Sorry, but you're going to be charged for not even being in the building." It's even tougher to say it to a friend, which your clients are. Friends are meant to be understanding of each other, and I really try to be. But when I screw up a session time, I always give a free session the next time. So when they screw up a session time, I expect similar respect. It's part of the training deal; someone has to lose money and you will need to be ultra-professional and consistent about determining who.

After sixteen years of trial and error, here's how I handle the cancellation policy. Every trainer is different about this, so you can ask others for their ideas. But this is how I handle it. I'm very up front when I meet new clients. Usually I'll explain that I don't like charging money for no reason. That's not the point of my job. But I'll talk them through several scenarios about what it looks like when I do charge and how I make the decision. You woke up with food poisoning? I'm not charging you. Your kid had to go to the hospital overnight? No problem. You were on the way out the door and every pipe in your house exploded? Totally get it.

But when people forget about me, book something else on top of our session, decide that they would rather sleep in, have a hangover, their kid has math homework due, they realized they can't get their grocery shopping done if they come to our session, something comes up at work, they have a repairman coming between 10am and 4pm, etc, I charge them. It's important that clients know that you are in the building specifically for them. When they reserve a time with you, no one else can reserve it. If you cancel for something avoidable and we don't charge you, it wastes our time, money, and scheduling space for another person.

Being sick is one of the most complicated reasons for cancelling. Because people don't want to lose their cash, they're likely to show up with colds, pneumonia, and god knows what else. Tell your clients right off the bat that if they're sick, please give you as much notice as possible and then stay home. No one wants diseases in the gym, and exercising with things like flu, strep, or covid is bad for your heart and body anyway. I had one client call me five minutes before our session and say, "Hey, Mia, I have conjunctivitis in both eyes, did you want me to come in? I don't want to get charged for the session."

FUCK. NO. STAY THE FUCK AWAY FROM ME. I don't even want you in Massachusetts.

However! There's a flip side to this. I have also had many times where someone says, "Hey, I've had this cold for a week and it's still lingering, so sorry I can't make it in." Meanwhile, I'm already sitting there waiting for them to show up. That's bullshit. You've been sick for a week, you can cancel me more than ten minutes in advance. When someone does that to me, I do charge them.

People will fight you. No one likes to lose money and everyone thinks their reason for not showing up is a good one. So do your best to set clear boundaries in the beginning about what you do and don't think is acceptable. People often think that their personal trainer gets paid by the gym to be in the building. That's not how it works. Trainers only get paid per session that they do, and a full-time trainer has a very tightly-packed schedule. I often have seven or eight sessions back-to-back with no break. (Because I want to give people the time they want, and also don't want to have unpaid hours in my schedule.)

If you show up late, I usually can't stay after the session to make up the time. If you ask me at 9am to move our 10am session to 2pm, I usually can't do that. I'll try, of course. But usually not. One woman I used to train would come in late and then be angry that I couldn't stay for the full hour. She'd say, "Well, I wouldn't have come if I knew it wasn't going to be worth my time." And what about my time, Karen? What about the time of the person who trains immediately after you?

This last part is important. Clients, especially if they're new to training, often don't realize that being flaky affects more than just the trainer. If I stay late for you because you arrived late, I'll be starting the next session late. If someone cancels their 10am at the last minute, anyone else who would have wanted that 10am spot is also affected. I hate that even more than I hate my own time being wasted. Giving people the workouts and times they want is my top priority. The worst situation is if someone special-requests the 10am, I free it up for them by moving another person to a different slot, and then the first person cancels. If I've moved another session to make room for your request, and then you don't show up for it? WHEW does that make me mad.

You might be wondering why I would move one client for another. If someone already had the spot, then they already had the spot, right? Yes and no. A personal trainer's schedule is complicated and delicately woven. It's not easy to get thirty, forty, or even fifty people booked into a calendar every week. Many people can only train at certain times of day, and a girl only has so many 8am sessions to offer. This means that when there is competition for a certain time, I have to ask my more flexible clients if another time might work for them, so that I can try to fit as many people in at the times they need. If you're not willing to play scheduling Jenga all the time, you won't be able to keep full-time hours as a trainer. Even people who book regular slots with me every week have to change them at least once in a while. You'll get really good at tracking client vacations/holidays, learning people's habits, and keeping tabs on open slots that people want. (e.g. I have a client who always wants 10am. When a 10am opens, I immediately text her.) I work the hardest at scheduling my most dedicated people. If someone turns out to be flaky, I won't try nearly as hard to fit in their preferred times, because they haven't proven to me that they'll show up for them.

Shuffling your schedule around is part of the job. But a reminder: even if a client is flexible, no one wants to feel like they're getting moved around constantly. It makes them feel like they're not as important as your other clients. I try very hard to alternate which clients I ask to switch times. You don't want to inconvenience the same person all the time.

You will need to learn how to discuss money, payments, and cancellations without being weird about it. My best advice is to decide ahead of time what you will and won't put up with, and then be clear with your clients about those boundaries. Tell them when you're going to charge them for a session and be ready to explain your reasoning if they ask. In the end, people are usually cool, especially if you make efforts to be cool as well. It's rare that someone gives me a hard time about the twenty-four hour rule. In fact, most people usually say, "I understand this is a late cancel, feel free to charge me," even if they are sick or something unavoidable came up, which is extremely kind. I still follow my rules though, in order to be consistent. So even with their permission to charge, I don't always do it. I'd rather maintain goodwill when I can.

I did lose one good client over my rigidity re: the cancellation policy. But I stand by the reason I charged him. President Obama was in town and Cambridge was completely locked down (this was well-known info in advance). Traffic was a mess everywhere. I got up two hours early to be sure I could get there on time for his session. About thirty minutes before the session, he emailed to tell me that traffic was a mess and he didn't want to bother driving through. I let him know I'd be charging him. He got super mad. I gave him a phone call and we had a civil chat about it. I explained that I had made the effort to get there early because of the circumstances and I expected him to do the same. He said he better understood my reasoning but didn't agree with it and that was our last session. It happens.

With clients you really like, I always immediately try to intervene when there's a potential problem. If they sound annoyed, I give them a call rather than emailing. If I see them in the gym, I'm going to ask if they have a minute to go over things in person. A good life lesson is that talking with voices is always better than talking with typing, especially when it's a potentially contentious situation. Don't fight with anyone by text message or email. You never know how your words are being received, because they can't hear your tone through text. And don't be insanely stubborn unless you don't care about losing the person. Keeping a client is usually better for you than standing your ground. That being said, here's an example of me going one hundred percent against that advice.

You will have entitled clients who expect that you will always operate on their time, because they're paying for it. These people are awful to work with and do not respect a single thing about the cancellation policy no matter how well you explain it. Those clients don't stay with me for long, because I go from zero to crazy bitch in a nanosecond when someone wastes my time and doesn't care.

One man that I worked with was always a little bit cutting towards me. He would make snide comments to critique various parts of how I work and train, like being a "standard fussy woman" and asking me to always be ten minutes early so we could start his warm-up together before his session officially began. (What the fuck.) I didn't like training him, but I was a relatively new trainer and not in a position to give up his sessions either.

One Wednesday morning, he didn't show up at 7am. At 7:15, I called him, as I would call any client to make sure they're ok and see if they're coming in. He answered the phone—I swear to God this is true—by hissing, "Hello? Mia? How dare you call me during my golf game? I am WITH people right now."

If you just laughed out loud, so did I.

I said, as politely as I could, "Well, sorry to interrupt, Greg, but I was expecting to be training you at 7am today so I was just checking in."

"We aren't booked for 7am. It's so disrespectful of you to be calling me right now."

"We were booked for 7am. I'd be happy to forward you the email where you confirmed the time." (I fucking love receipts.)

"Sure, go ahead and send that. Goodbye," and he hung up on me.

Boy. I have NEVER been so excited to dive into my computer, immediately pull up the email from him which had the exact date and time of the session, and smash that Forward button. Like and subscribe, folks!

He never acknowledged the email or the booking. Instead, he began sending email after email, raging about how he thought we were friends, raging about how disrespectful I am, raging about how greedy I am that I wanted to charge him $70 for the session when I should be more understanding about how busy he is. (Never forget that the more wrong someone is, the angrier they get.)

There is an interesting part of the story here, which is a perfect example of the client/trainer friendly relationship getting spicy. Greg owned an apartment in Paris and had let me stay there prior to all this happening. His view, as I learned from his appalling emails, was that because he loaned me his apartment, he was exempt forever from my training boundaries, including cancellations. My view was (and is) that a client offering a gift to me does it of their own accord and cannot use it as a bounty over our professional work. As I said, I always try to be as understanding as possible, but I don't make professional exemptions for people who have given me gifts, even luxe ones. First of all, my professional standards aren't for sale. Second of all, there is no need or obligation to offer me gifts ever, so it would be disrespectful to my clients who don't to that for me to give favoritism to the clients who do. Third of all, it is a slippery slope to "pay back" the gift with free or discounted sessions. How many missed-sessions-for-golf should I forgive before I've paid back an apartment in Paris? I believe Greg would have said all of them. That's not how this works, no matter how fucking cool it was that he let me use their place. I have been extremely lucky to stay in many client's vacation homes in my career and none of them have ever expected what Greg expected from it.

Anyway, Greg and I met in person to discuss the situation, only after his wife forced him to. What was that meeting like? Imagine a three-year-old discovering that it's their sibling's birthday, not theirs. That was Greg. Our "discussion" ended with him standing up, smashing two hands down on the tabletop, red-faced, bulging eyes, leaning towards me threateningly, screaming, "HOW DARE YOU FORCE ME TO WORK WITH ANOTHER TRAINER BY ACTING LIKE THIS?!"

I couldn't help it. I laughed out loud. He entered an apocalypse state. When he finally stopped screaming, panting heavily like a stampeding wildebeest, I said, "Greg. Hold on. What do you mean force you to get a new trainer? Of course you need a new trainer. You...thought that we were going to train again after this?" and he said, "YES OF COURSE. Just on MY terms, not yours."

This sent me through the stratosphere. I burst out laughing and he stormed out of the building. I never saw him again, though he continued to email me insulting tirades for a while.

I refunded his money in the end because I was tired of him screaming at me. And, as I tried to tell him, it's not about the money for me. Yes, of course I lost out on the session pay. But I'm not greedy for forty fucking dollars. I care that he never acknowledged any part of inconveniencing me or wasting my time. If, when I called him during his golf game, he had said, "Oh my god, I totally forgot I was going to be away this week, I'm so sorry," I would have answered, "It's no problem, thanks for saying that. See you Friday?" It would have been over. And I can say that confidently, because it's happened hundreds of times with dozens of other clients. Of course people make scheduling mistakes! If it doesn't happen often, all I usually ask for is an apology. But to be so rude to me when I have your email confirming your appointment time, plus shaming me for contacting you during your golf game? Yeah, no. That doesn't work for me.

It's one of my favorite stories to tell new trainers, because there is a thick river of entitlement that can come along with providing services to people. When people pay a lot of money for a service, they often think of you as The Help, someone who can be controlled by money and bent to conform to their whim. I've had plenty of clients with whom I always felt the hierarchy. They were the rich, powerful, and important one, and I was the gym employee. Greg didn't care about my training abilities nearly as much as he cared about controlling me. It infuriated him (and I suspect my gender didn't help) that I pushed back against him instead of crumpling beneath his rich fingertip. When you work as a trainer, remember that the terms of service are yours. Yes, you should do everything you can to be accommodating. But in the end, you determine the terms, and don't let them be bought.

So where should you draw the final line on charging for cancellations? It's up to you, or possibly the gym you work in. Some places do an automatic account withdrawal at exactly the twenty-four hour mark, and it doesn't matter the circumstances the client finds themselves in. Others, the trainer has full control over entering all the sessions they completed, so they can adjust the calendar as they please. That's how our gym operates, because people shouldn't be penalized if they have so much diarrhea they can't stand up without it cascading down their leg. I certainly wouldn't want to work out if I had the Mississippi River forging a new path through my pants. The more experience you get, the more you'll understand which cancellation fights to pick and which ones to let go. I promise, most people are cool about it. Most people are not Greg.

There are some other tangential business difficulties that might come up for you, especially if you work at a large corporate chain like I did. I lost some clients over the years because of some repulsive gym managers and some real shit behavior by the corporate offices of the company. As a trainer at a corporate gym, you represent the brand, yet you have absolutely no control over corporate policies. It can get sticky. People got upset when they had membership dues increases, when repairs weren't being made on the gym, when the temperature in the gym was poorly regulated, when they would email a manager and not hear back from them, etc. It always made me feel bad; we couldn't do much about these things but I could feel my clients gradually losing interest in the gym because of them. The best you can do is talk with your GM about the issues, but recognize that not everything in the gym is under your control. People might love training with you but might not love the gym you're at. If that happens, let them leave if they want, but hold onto their contact info. If you ever change gyms, you might be able to bring them back.

There are two other parts of the business side of things that I want to go over. The first is handling the people who want your time and expertise for free. These people are everywhere. They are the members at the gym who don't want to pay for personal training but want the trainers to give them advice and supervise their sets. They are friends and family who want you to write programs for them, as if you could dash it off in five seconds. They are the people you meet in bars, restaurants, and at networking events who want your thoughts on their workouts. I once was eating alone at a bar, wearing my Personal Trainer sweatshirt. One of the servers, who was not my server, interrupted my meal four times to ask my opinion on various parts of his running training. Good god, bro. Please let me eat my snap pea risotto. I always try to be nice to people but also don't want to spend my entire quiet lunch discussing your fartlek intervals. I am sure this happens to doctors and physical therapists, too. The minute someone at a party finds out I'm a personal trainer, they dive into a play-by-play of their daily workout routine. It makes me want to launch myself into the sun.

As always, it's up to you how much you want to give of yourself for free. I recommend that you give a lot—especially when you're new in the field and need to build a name for yourself—but that you set some boundaries (are you sensing a theme here). People have no idea how long it takes to write an individualized program. They also have no idea that a question like, "Hey, do you have any advice on what to do for legs?" is both hilarious and meaningless. (People will ask you this constantly.) I will always answer questions for friends and family but I will not write training programs for anyone who is not a paying client. Not my best friend, not my parents.

And, by the way, I also don't write extensive training programs for my clients (even if they do offer to pay). If you have just a few clients a week, sure, you can do this. I have about fifty-five regular clients. Writing and maintaining fifty-five complete programs would be a full-time job by itself, without any gym time together. Can't do it. Instead, I teach my clients how to program themselves in between our sessions.

My biggest pet peeve on this topic is when people ask me for a program to do while they're on vacation/away for the summer/post-surgical, etc. I used to be perfectly happy to do this, until I discovered that 99.9% of people never even look at the program I send. Writing up a week's worth of workouts would take me forty-five minutes to an hour. A whole summer of workouts would take a few hours. To have people repeatedly say, "Oh, no, I didn't get to any of it," was depressing and angering, so I stopped doing it. Now, when people ask, I offer to send them a list of exercises that I'd like them to work on, but I don't write the program. It only takes me a few minutes and then it's up to them to create their sets and reps.

The final thing I want to discuss about the business side of things is about working within your own professional lane. It's super common for people to think of trainers as a one-stop shop for all of their health woes. People will come in wanting your opinion on their kidney stones, gout, concussions, blood results, imaging results, etc. I swear, you'll start to feel like a little personal Minute Clinic. A pregnant client of mine was present at the finish line of the Boston Marathon bombing, and the first place she went after it happened? To me, to ask if I thought her baby was damaged by the catastrophic noise level and trauma. (Her baby eventually came out beautifully.)

The whole situation is understandable. Great personal trainers are well-versed in the human body, and our clients trust us. It's easier to get an appointment with your trainer than with your doctor, and more convenient than going to see a physical therapist. For trainers, it's easy to sink deeply into the feeling that you can help your clients with a lot of bodily problems (because you can). And it's easy to sink into the feeling that exercise might be the solution for the majority of those problems (because it definitely could be). Still, your entire role as a trainer is to get a good understanding of the person in front of you and then provide safe exercises for their body as you currently understand it. That's it. That means if the body in front of you is changing, you have no place diagnosing it, recommending medications, offering diet/meal plans, etc. The best you can do here is to give extremely general knowledge that any health-centered person would know, and then refer out to the proper expert.

You will get clients over the years who come down with all kinds of diseases and strange symptoms and ailments, and you'll hear about all of those in detail. This does not make you a doctor. People tend to lump food and fitness together, so you'll hear a ton about people's eating habits and nutrition. This does not make you a nutritionist. And over the years, you'll be responsible for caring for a lot of injured joints. This does not make you a physical therapist. Sometimes clients are annoyed by this (no one wants to add more appointments into their days), and might ask to do more and more sessions with you to try and fix their body with strength training. More sessions are great because they equal more money for you, but responsibility to your client is more important. Even if your client gets irritated with you, do not work out of your lane, and refer people out when they need help instead of assuming you can do it yourself.

That said, sometimes more educated health professionals are dead. fucking. wrong. about exercise. Doctors have said some whack-ass shit to my clients. Things like never squat again because it's bad for your back; stop running because it's bad for your knees; pick up swimming after age fifty because it's the only safe exercise; rest and ice injuries. These things are false. There is no research to support them.

It can be tough when a doctor gives your client bad advice, because it's a doctor. Their word is tops in our society. Unfortunately, they usually know very little about fitness. I will tactfully push back when a client brings me doctor garbage, because I want my client to be working with the best possible information. I will also offer to talk with the physician personally, even though I know that no doctor will ever bother to find the time for me. Either way, I'll still try to explain the actual science and research to my client. I won't overstep my bounds into practicing medicine for my clients, but that means I also won't let medical practitioners overstep their bounds into fitness. If a client comes to you with some wild tales from a doctor, don't be afraid to trust your education and hold your ground on it. Ultimately it'll be your client's decision who to believe, but you'll have done your job.

The next chapter digs into this exact issue of collaborative care, because it's a critical question for our industry. But for now, remember that, even when you're sure of what's going on, you cannot throw out medical opinions to your clients. I will often say things like, "This looks like [x] injury that I've seen in clients before but..." or "Generally, biceps tendon pain is secondary to rotator cuff problems but..." and then the end of the sentence is going to be, "you should go see a doctor or physical therapist to get an accurate assessment." Make sure you always tack that part on. You never want someone coming back to you with an accusation or worse.

When people trust you, they'll take your advice very seriously, so make sure it's advice that you're qualified to give. Even when it *is* advice you're qualified to give, people are liable to twist it around, so hone your communication skills to be razor sharp. I had one client ask me for general information about losing weight, which I gave her. We trained for a while and then she stopped for no given reason. She came back a year later, spitting mad, because she had been diagnosed with a condition which was affecting her fertility. She hissed at me, "Guess your thoughts that I was drinking too much didn't have anything to do with anything," demanded a refund on all of our training, and stormed away.

I was dumbfounded, and my feelings were hurt. We had never talked about the reason that she wanted to lose weight, or her fertility at all, but she was still furious with me. I didn't deserve her rage, but if I'd been a more experienced trainer when we met, I would have spent more time in our original conversation finding out why she was so intent on losing weight. We might have edged towards the fertility question, at which point I could have redirected the conversation into places where I can offer sound advice. (Exercise can benefit fertility independently of weight loss, and I would have loved to share that with her and point her towards a fertility doctor who could tell her more.)

People with body insecurity and pain will pin a lot of shit on you in this career. They'll hold you responsible for deep-seated body issues that you have absolutely nothing to do with and no ability to solve. I knew my infertile client wasn't actually angry with me. She was bereft at not being able to conceive and looking for any kind of outlet to release that grief. People's bodies are the most personal thing they own, and you can never overestimate the emotional charge we all carry about them (especially women). But you don't want to be a punching bag either. This is why you always need to be trying to understand the entire person and the entire situation in front of you. A high EQ and excellent communication skills will help everyone. I obviously did not refund any of the training we did together, and she didn't ask me again. But in other situations, you will need to let the money go and operate with compassion for a person who needs help. People always have shit going on, and your ongoing effort will benefit both of you in the long run.

Working as a personal trainer will teach you a ton about business. I'm extremely comfortable now asking for money, refusing to work if I'm not being paid, believing in the valuable service that I know I can offer, etc. I don't apologize for being expensive. And, in turn, I've become more empathetic over the years, more interested in helping my clients succeed overall than in taking their money at every opportunity. (This is admittedly easier to develop when you're not a new trainer, desperate for every single session you can get.) All of these skills will be tested immediately upon starting work, so a wise new trainer will consider their boundaries and practice money talk before it ever comes up with a client.

Next up? Collaborative care, especially with physical therapists. If you want to enter the personal trainer-physical therapist coliseum to witness the battles, turn the page. Otherwise, skip straight to my thoughts on the industry, where the rest of the tea is steeping.

TL;DR:

1) Get comfortable talking about money, and don't be afraid to ask for money when it is owed to you.

2) Be extremely clear with your clients about when you will apply the twenty-four hour cancellation policy and when you will not. Remember that no matter how many rules you make, there will always be exceptions.

3) Always stand up for yourself and your right to be paid, but if you're not sure, then you're better off erring on the side of not charging your client than charging them. Sometimes diplomacy is worth more.

4) Don't let people boss you around, mistreat you, or disrespect your time just because they're paying you money. Even when you're a new trainer and need cash, you shouldn't let yourself be used, taken advantage of, or treated like shit.

5) Remember a trainer's scope of practice. People might offer to pay you for nutrition advice, physical therapy, or even extra training in order to treat their medical issue. If you aren't sure, refer out. Even the best doctors in the world are regularly flummoxed. You do not need to pretend to know everything that's ever been known about the human body.

Chapter Ten: Collaborative Care

The sad truth of this job is that you will not be able to fix everyone. For one, you won't have time. It takes years of work to get most people into a place where they can independently sustain good health habits. You only have forty hours in a week.

For another, plenty of people aren't in your scope. They don't need you, they need physical therapy, medical interventions, or surgery.

Other people won't like you. They won't like your personality, your teaching style, your methods of communication, your body, or just you in general.

Some will ask your advice and then immediately argue with or discredit it. Others will ask for your advice over and over again, and then defy it over and over again, because, as Jan says in The Office, they want you to slowly collapse in on yourself like a dying star. I've worked with some people who have been asking my advice for a decade and still haven't taken it.

This work can make you feel insane. Why would so many people ask for your help and then not take it? You're an expert on the subject with a strong desire to help guide and teach people. They're paying you to hear what you think! And then don't care what you think! Wtf. It feels like a personal affront when someone isn't interested in your services. Why don't they want to work with me? I'm incredible! Mia's Magic Exercises for all! I can fix you!

Ego, ego, ego. Human psychology is a deep subject and it's not all about you. If you aren't getting through to someone, help them find someone else who might be able to.

Step one of collaborative care: let go of the idea that you are the only one who can help everyone. I can't tell you how many people who work in healthcare believe that they are the Be-All-End-All of feeling better.

Our trainer egos can get large. There is a certain power that comes with having the ability to heal people (as every cocky physical therapist and dismissive surgeon knows), and effective trainers are not immune to it. We get aggravated when people don't listen to us. We always think we know exactly what they need to do. I'm at the point where I absentmindedly watch strangers walk down the street and imagine all of the foot and ankle exercises I want to give them. I stare at people having a difficult time reaching the bottom shelf at the grocery store and instantly want to get them in my clutches. I have been known to subtly start a conversation and try to work some tips into it. I'm not proud of it. But sometimes I can't resist. I want to help people so badly, and I know through my bones that if people partook in regular, good-quality movement, the vast majority would feel way better and be way healthier. Movement heals, and trainers know this. It's why most of us became trainers in the first place.

But movement doesn't ALWAYS heal. You won't always have the answer. No one has all the answers. You'll need to keep your eyes open for when it's appropriate to refer your client out to a different professional. You're not the gatekeeper of a person's health or the only person who knows what's going on. I know this seems obvious but you wouldn't believe how many trainers refuse to send their clients to someone else. They just keep pounding away with the same exercises. (Same with physical therapists. Physicians tend to be a little better.) You don't want to send every client to the doctor every time something twangs in their shoulder. But if they've got a pain they can't shake for months, it's not likely that more overhead presses are gonna be the cure for it.

First step in collaborative care is to cultivate good relationships with some physical therapists. Some injuries do need movement to heal, but it might not be *your* type of movement that the injury needs. You'll refer people out when a body part needs more specialized attention than you can give. Developing a great symbiotic relationship with a few PTs is awesome because you'll have people you trust to take care of your clients, and those PTs will refer you when their patients graduate from specialized care.

Just be aware that you're going to have to battle some awful physical therapists on the way to finding the good ones.

The relationship between personal trainers and physical therapists is ROUGH. It shouldn't be, it's completely fucking insane that the two lines of work don't get along perfectly, but it is nonetheless. So let's talk about that for a second, because I'm hoping that some physical therapists will be reading this.

Physical therapists are notorious for thinking that personal trainers are reckless, under-educated, and constantly putting their clients at risk of injury. Personal trainers are notorious for thinking that physical therapy is too conservative, palliative, and a general waste of time. If you surf rehab Instagram, TikTok, Threads, or Twitter, you'll see an infinite number of comments from one group shitting on the other for not knowing what they're talking about. It's entertaining but also frustrating.

Who's right? Well, go get a fresh cup of tea cuz I've got your answers here.

I spent a good eight years of my training career telling anyone who would listen that physical therapy was a bunch of garbage. I argued that the movements they asked for were too small to make a difference in a body that works in one giant unit of harmony all the time. That it didn't make sense to have a major surgery, then sit with an electrical stimulator on your shoulder for ten minutes twice a week, and think that that would heal anything.

I was half-right. I thought physical therapy was garbage because the only physical therapy I'd ever had was garbage. If your physical therapy consists of electrical stimulation, followed by ice, followed by heat, and then you get sent home? That's garbage. I had that style of PT after my first ankle surgery. If you're in the clinic for twenty minutes and your provider is seeing three other patients at the same time? Garbage. I had that after herniating several discs in my lower back. Appointments should be an hour and although most PTs are forced to see multiple people at once, if it's more than two, change clinics or go at quieter times. If the PT isn't watching you do everything, giving corrections, and answering questions, they're not helping you. And if you're not being physically challenged in every PT session just like a strength training workout? Garbage. I had that for disc pain in my mid-back. I ended up rehabbing all of those things by myself, and deciding that physical therapy was useless.

I was half right, but I was also half-wrong. (Or maybe more than half wrong...) I thought that PT movements were too small to matter when you consider the way the human body works as a whole. Dead wrong. It took me eight years of work in this field to realize that you must be able to individualize movements in every joint. Yes, the body works as a whole of its parts. But if the individual parts can't move independently, then the whole is compromised. Every part that can't move well by itself is a threat to the other parts of the system.

For example, a sprint uses all of the giant leg muscles. So I always focused on training the quads, hams, and glute max to get faster. I never understood how doing tiny glute medius training could really help with sprints. I just saw it as an accessory. But the tiny glute medius is responsible for transferring force smoothly from the legs to the trunk, via pelvic stability. When it's too weak to keep up, the hips will sway side-to-side every time the person's feet hit the ground. The person will experience energy leaks on every stride. The lower back and knees will have to do more than their usual to stabilize the body, and the faster they're going, the more overtime everyone needs to put in. So ignoring glute medius (and others) while sprinting makes you slower and more vulnerable to injury. Yuck. Optimization of the small stabilizers is what allows the giant muscles to do their work at full blast. That's the information I didn't understand, and it's what physical therapy is the best for.

You might be wondering why it took me eight years as a highly-educated and experienced trainer to realize this. The first reason is that although I knew it on a superficial level, I hadn't intellectually dug deeply enough. I simply hadn't assigned the stabilizers enough credit as workhorses. I would train them in conjunction with the big muscles, but never on their own. The more biomechanics I learned, the more I realized all of the impressive ways that the body can compensate for poor stability. It's so seamless, it took me a long time to be able to spot and correct those compensations. The second reason is that I needed more time in my own body as it aged to understand how aging was happening in other people. When I was twenty-three, a client asked me what I did when I had injuries. I literally responded with, "I don't really get injured." LMAO. At the time, I thought it was because my training was so supreme that I was immune to injury. It wasn't. I just had a very young body which was also well-taken care of. That can take you a good distance, but not forever. As I learned more about my own body and the ways my own training evolved through the years, it became easier to understand other people's bodies and the way their training needed to evolve.

My feelings on physical therapy changed completely as soon as I had a good PT, my friend Luke. He convinced me to come in against my will for my rampant lower back pain. He raised his eyebrows at my inability to flex forward or sideways. He asked me to show him my thoracic rotation, which was, in all seriousness, about three degrees in each direction. He tested my glute medius strength which was like pushing your hand through a bowl of jello. Luke was like, are you fucking kidding me? Your whole spine is rigid, your hips are for shit, you do high-impact exercise, and you're wondering why you have a ton of back pain? Have you ever done a single rotational exercise in your life? (No.) Do you have a single muscle fiber in your glutes? (No.) Have you ever tried bending and straightening your spine? (No.) And then he kicked my ass. I was like what the fuck is this physical therapy? Where's my heating pad? Why are these squats making me want to sob? How dare you point out that I have no hip muscles? RUDE LUKE GO WORK WITH SOMEONE ELSE. I KNOW WHAT I'M DOING.

Narrator's voice: She did not know what she was doing.

Physical therapy is physical; it's supposed to be work. After spine PT with Luke, I added intense mobility work to my repertoire. Teaching my spine how to rotate, flex, and extend, and then strengthening my hips and butt times a thousand was life-changing. After five herniated discs, lots of degeneration, a flat spine, and ten years of constant back pain, I got rid of it completely. It wasn't fast—it took two to three years of consistent work—but I could feel little improvements on the way. I give Luke lots of credit for picking me up and placing me on the right path. That's what a great PT (and what great trainers) will do. They identify the correct path, and then show you how to go down it yourself. Because they won't always be there in person to kick your ass.

Since then, I've had several great PTs but the best one is Emily. She kicked my ass on day one, was super attentive to my problems and questions, and she referred me out when she thought she needed help with my case instead of assuming she could fix it herself with enough time. Zero ego. It turned out I did need surgery, and my outcome was phenomenal. I would never have gone to see a surgeon without her. You need a humble PT who respects your injury, understands your injury, but isn't scared of your injury. I'll talk more about how to find a good PT a little later in this chapter.

So I've personally become very pro-physical therapy, but only with a limited number of trusted PTs. I still distrust a lot of them. I've been burned by too many assholes in the industry and I know they're still everywhere, lying in wait for their next opportunity to take a dump on the next unsuspecting personal trainer.

Let me start by saying that even when I didn't believe in physical therapy, I always wanted to talk to my clients' physical therapists to coordinate care of complex cases. I wanted to know what my clients were or weren't allowed to do, and I wanted to know the therapist's opinion on the path forward. So I've often reached out when my clients are in physical therapy, hoping to connect with their therapist to make a plan.

Over sixteen years of calling physical therapists to talk about clients, here's what I've noticed. Female PTs have a 100% success rate of getting back to me, almost always by phone. They help me review my client's case and make sure that I have a good understanding of my role in the process. They respect my work as a trainer without making me feel like I'm dumb or dangerous. Often they want me to scale back my client's work more than I would like to, but I can deal with that. I've never had a female PT be condescending to me.

Male PTs? I almost never hear back, and when I do, it's gone pretty badly. One guy, Jason, told my post-hip-replacement client that he would absolutely not get on the phone with me. Why not? He said,

"Because I have a doctorate, and she wouldn't understand the work that I'm doing with you. It's not worth trying to explain it to her."

Along with being stunned, you're probably wondering what the sensational and complicated work he was doing with her was. It was sitting to a chair and standing up again. It was walking sideways with a band around her ankle. It was calf raises. Blistering academic work, if you ask me, but what do I know? I'm just tootling around, wishing I had an understanding of bending your knees and straightening them again.

Another PT, Josh (what is it with the J names?), did call me back, and then screamed at me on the phone for several minutes. He opened the conversation aggressively, with, "Good, I'm glad you answered, because I need to talk to you." I was taken aback, but said, "Yes, good! I want to talk to you too, that's why I reached out." And then I didn't get to say much else, because he launched into this:

"What you're doing with Ellen is extremely dangerous and irresponsible. Are you kidding me? She's doing bear crawls all over the gym? Are you fucking kidding me? She has a stapled shoulder and back pain and that's what you're doing with her?"

Me, attempting to calm him down, "No, that's not what I'm doing with her. She must have mistakenly reported something to you. Why are you swearing at me?"

"Because you deserve this. You're the reason that Ellen has to keep coming back to PT. You're destroying her. If you can't understand why she should be doing something like a side plank instead of bear crawls, do not train her again. You are going to permanently injure her."

Me, "You...want me to assign...side planks...to someone with a reconstructed shoulder?" (Side planks are notoriously difficult and/

or painful for people with long-standing shoulder issues and reconstructions. This recommendation was legitimately insane.)

Josh, "I want you to do what I'm telling you to do, or do not touch her again."

Me, "Well, this has been a pleasant conversation. Thank you so much for calling."

Josh, *hangs up*

The rudeness of this conversation was unreal. But what bothered me the most is that Josh never asked me a single thing about my experience or my sessions with Ellen. If he was really this concerned about her, he would have wanted as much information about our work as possible. It would be entirely reasonable to discover that a trainer was new and might accidentally be giving ill-advised work. Great opportunity to offer guidance. But he didn't. He didn't ask about my time in the field, my education, or if I have experience with older populations. He also didn't ask me a single thing about her. He didn't ask me to list the exercises we do most often, or how she responds to them. He didn't even clarify if what she had reported to him was accurate. He just took an express train straight to Grand Cuntral Station and got off, flapping his junk around.

This is the kind of shit that divides physical therapists and personal trainers and makes each one a hater of the other. And it's not unique to me. Physical therapists shit on personal trainers and vice versa all the time. You'll hear it at conferences and workshops, and you'll hear it via third parties, like when a physical therapist tells my client that I'm too stupid to understand what his PhDickhead brain is doing.

Most of the time, this distrust is based on a huge misunderstanding of what each person actually does in their workspace. And that misunderstanding is compounded by relying on our mutual client to accurately relay information between us. This is one reason why I always try to talk to PTs directly. Clients are extremely bad at relaying information. They often can't remember things precisely, and often don't have a great knowledge of their own body. This combination can lead to a report which is full of inaccuracies.

My client Ellen letting Josh know that we do bear crawls all the time? When Josh and I had that conversation, it had been years since Ellen and I practiced any floor crawling. But she reported it as if it were recently. Another client of mine once told her PT that we did box jumps together. He sent me an email to tell me that box jumping was extremely dangerous for her and to stop. She and I had done box jumps exactly one time, when she specifically asked me to try some because she saw other people doing them and was curious if she had the ability. (If you're wondering, I will never say no to something a client wants to try. So we did a safe set-up to show yes, she could box jump. And yes, she was super proud of herself. And no, we never did them again.)

A third client of mine, fifty-five years old, told his doctor that we "regularly get his heart rate up to 200 beats per minute" during sessions.

You should have seen my face. I was like, "You told him WHAT?!"

That doctor told my client that we needed to stop that kind of work immediately. When my client mentioned this to me, I said, "Dave. We literally never get your heart rate anywhere close to that." And he said, "Well, it feels like it."

(scream emoji)

Here's why this happens. What clients usually remember best about their sessions is, ironically, not the stuff they do most often. This is because of how memory works. When asked to recall details about a given experience, our brains don't call up boring, rote memories of that experience. Boring, rote memories get filtered out. What we retain is uncommon or surprising memories, so the stuff a client remembers about exercise is the stuff that's unusual, extra challenging, or most fun.

When doctors or physical therapists ask my clients what they do in the gym, they generally just list off a few memorable things that come to mind. Things like bear crawls, box jumps, or super high heart rate work—the uncommon stuff. To an experienced health provider, those reports can raise all kinds of red flags. But anyone with a brain and a desire to provide care for their patient would call me to hear my version of the story. Unfortunately, related to how women are disrespected in strength and conditioning, my experience has largely been male providers assuming the worst about me and then trying to verbally tackle me into behaving.

Special shout-out here to Kevin and (a different) Josh, two male PTs who were wonderful to me, called me back, had in-depth conversations about our clients, and made sure they understood what I was doing and I understood what they were doing. Not all men! ;)

In spite of being yelled at by the men except for Kevin and Different Josh, I am now strongly pro-physical therapy personally and professionally. I often refer patients out, and I keep a list of good PTs that I trust and who trust in my work as well. You should keep a list like this too.

But the real question to ask here is more macro: Why on earth would two fields, which highly overlap each other, with nearly identical goals, and nearly identical work, and who naturally create a logical bridge to move patients from one to the next as they get healthier, hate each other so much? We should be perfect partners. I have two explanations.

My first theory as to why therapists and trainers don't get along is because of perspective. Physical therapists only ever see relatively injured bodies, and trainers only ever see relatively healthy bodies. It can be like a glass-half-full thing, where a trainer and a PT see the same person but arrive at totally opposite conclusions about that person. Neither is right or wrong, it happens simply because of our natural work biases. A physical therapist tends to see all the imbalances and question marks that could be causing an issue. A trainer tends to see all the parts working beautifully and wants to capitalize on those things. Both are valid.

Take someone who wants to learn a deadlift. PTs are not generally big fans of deadlifting. The only deadlifters they see are the ones who got hurt enough to need physical therapy. They might tell their client to avoid deadlifting, because they'll get hurt. Personal trainers are generally big fans of deadlifting. They only see deadlifters who get strong as hell from it. They might tell their client to definitely deadlift, because they'll get strong.

The truth, as always, lies in the middle. Deadlifting is right for many people, but not all. Avoiding deadlifting is right for many people, but not all. This brings us directly back to my argument that trainers and PTs MUST prioritize the patient in front of them and see their needs directly. Therapists need to remember that not everything causes injury. Trainers need to remember that some things can cause injury. This change alone would improve trainer/therapist relationships.

My second theory as to why therapists and trainers don't get along is because of the health care system. (At least, in the United States.) There is a gap in care between physical therapy and personal training and our garbage health care/insurance system is the reason for it.

Insurance, when it comes to physical therapy, is bananas. A company who has never met us, evaluated us, or treated our injury, needs to grant permission to go to PT in the first place. We have to ask them for permission to get MRI's, genetic testing, and see specialists. If you're getting treated for your lower back, you can't get treated for your upper back at the same time. The PT needs a new authorization for that, even though it's the same fucking back and different parts of the same back affect each other. Insurance can also determine when your treatment is complete! Hooray! They decided you're better! They now refuse to pay for any further treatment. After that, as Taylor sings, you're on your own kid. You always have been.

It's beyond insane that we're all okay with this. And because of it, PT hands are often tied by red tape, which affects their care. This red tape, which is no one's fault except insurance companies and the governments who keep them in power, is responsible for a large part of the PT/PT divide.

The system sets people up for inadequate care. Let's say an adult tears an ACL. They get some prescribed number of physical therapy sessions and then insurance says hey, you should be healed by now. The person isn't healed, but the physical therapist has no power to do anything about it, so they release their patient back into the wild. This is deeply irresponsible on the part of insurance companies; this is the time when a patient needs the *most* supervision. The gap between a 70% healed injury and a 100% healed injury is MASSIVE. That patient, released early by insurance, still needs late-stage rehab. And they have two options for it. They can work out by themselves and hope it finishes the job. Or, if they can afford it, they can hire a personal trainer to help them finish the job.

Let's talk about the first option. Working out by yourself is already hard when you're healthy. But working out by yourself when you still have rehab to do? Super overwhelming and timing becomes a problem. Do you keep your normal workouts and add in rehab? You'll need twice the amount of time you usually take for exercise. Just go back to normal workouts? It feels like you're spending the whole time trying not to fly too close to the sun. Just do rehab? Doesn't feel like you're getting enough stimulus to improve things outside of the injury. Plus, if you do choose self-rehab, you're supposed to be building on the last exercises you were doing in the clinic. You're supposed to add weight, speed, impact, and change of direction—things that we rarely practice without a coach when healthy, let alone when still recovering. Do you know what the next progressions are, or how hard you can safely push yourself? Most have no idea.

So you go with the second option: get a personal trainer to help. We're great at weight, speed, impact, and change of direction work. But we're not trained in late-stage rehab, which involves knowing tissue tolerance, preventing backsliding, contraindicated exercises, warning signs of problems, understanding pain thresholds, being familiar with the research on the outcomes and expectations for any given injury, etc. It's not our field. But honestly, there aren't many physical therapists who are well-trained in late-stage rehab either. This is because they usually don't have patients getting that far before being discharged, or it's decided the patient doesn't need late-stage rehab at all, even if insurance would cover it. This is insane. A partial recovery isn't "good enough," though I've had so many PTs and doctors say that about my clients. Quality of life depends on speed, impact, and change of direction work, no matter someone's age or ability. Life happens at speed, with impact, and from multiple directions. There are physical therapists who are well-trained in performance rehab, and they're also often not covered by insurance because they knew better and got the fuck out of the clownshow. A private-practice physical therapist costs about twice as much as a personal trainer.

So patients are kicked out of PT, working out alone is indecipherable, and if they can even afford one, most personal trainers don't know late-stage rehab. Where does this all lead to? A country full of abandoned, partially-healed patients who have to hope they get better magically. This is the source of the whole enchilada: physical therapists who think personal trainers irresponsibly overstep their scope of practice (because we have to), and personal trainers who think that physical therapists never get their clients where they need to be before discharging them (because they have to).

It's trash, and it's all rooted in corporate greed. Keeping people sick is extremely profitable. In the meantime, we health professionals get pitted against each other for trying to pick up where the system leaves people off.

We need two things: first, a step-down in physical therapy, and second, personal training that's covered by insurance. The step-down would be like they have in hospitals for patients who are getting better but not ready to be discharged yet. I can't tell you how many people I've had over the years who came in saying, "I was doing physical therapy for [x], but it still hurts and I'd like to get it stronger." It's pretty much everyone who comes through the door. Some of that abysmal rate of return on physical therapy has to do with compliance, which is famously low in PT. (About 15% of patients do their physical therapy entirely as directed.) Some of it has to do with people running out of insurance coverage and stopping before they should stop. And some of it has to do with the fact that physical therapy never took them far enough to be comfortable in real life, which does require weight, speed, impact, and change of direction at every age and ability. All three situations need a step-down that's covered by insurance: A PersonalPhysicalTrainerTherapist. A Perphysapister, if you will. (Please don't.) Since we don't have Perphysapisters, we shit on each other, patients stay hurt, and someone else makes money.

The insane part is that our two fields should work together seamlessly. All we need is for physical therapy to go a little further down the performance road, for trainers to get a bit more education on late-stage rehab, and for insurance to cover some personal training to finish the job. Great physical therapy should merge beautifully into a training and performance program with a trainer. Right now, it's like there are two cliffs, and no one has ever bothered to build a solid bridge between them. The bridge that exists at the moment is a sketchy-ass rope bridge, with broken planks and all of these patients and clients crowded in the middle. They all need help. So someone's got to go get them and help them, and insurance won't let physical therapists do it. That means it's up to us.

In spite of what many physical therapists think, most trainers aren't arrogantly stomping across the bridge to get clients, without a care in the world about how many tendons they snap or menisci they lose on the way. Most trainers are picking their way across like oh shit, this person's shoulders have been hurting for years. I wonder if they can press. I wonder if they can pull. I wonder if they can go overhead. I wonder if their rotator cuff works. I wonder if they can tolerate repetitive strain. I'm not sure about any of it, so we have to try all of it. It would be easier to try if we had help from the clinicians who have already worked with them.

That's why I call my clients' physical therapists and get enraged when they don't call me back. Physical therapists, I know you're overworked, but please give more of a shit about your patients. I know most of them don't have personal trainers who call you. So please give at least one fuck about the patients who do have a trainer calling you, give a fuck about them having a positive outcome, and call me back. Stop acting like we're trash and start recognizing that we're trying to pick up pieces that you left off. Give us ten minutes of your time to point us in the right direction so that our client has a fighting chance of getting better. I guarantee that Josh and Jason, the PTs I mentioned earlier in the chapter, have shit-talked me to a coworker or two, and I don't deserve that.

And trainers, don't stop educating yourselves. You also have to give a fuck about your client's outcome. You haven't learned enough in your certifications. Learn anatomy and biomechanics more thoroughly. Pay attention to the injury rehab that your clients are doing when they're actively in physical therapy. Try to get in touch with the PT for guidance. Ask for copies of the exercises and stay abreast of where they're at. Ask a ton of questions. Read books. Read research. Learn about common causes for overuse injuries and learn to spot the warning signs for them. Ask for help. When you have a client in front of you with a pain or a problem that you don't know how to approach, you're better off working around it. They've got a weird knee going on? Focus on upper body, skip the squats, and see if you can do a shit-ton of hinging work instead. Tell your client that they and their weird knee need to go get a fresh PT prescription. And then stay on top of their weird-knee rehab, so that you can be better prepared for it when they get back. Plus, the next time you have someone with the same weird knee, you'll know what to do.

To both physical therapists and personal trainers, learn more about the other field. Meet people who work in those fields and get some cross-referral going on. There are plenty of bad physical therapists, and there are plenty of bad personal trainers. Keep track of the good ones. I've built a list of physical therapists who I am comfortable sending my clients to. And I have several physical therapist friends who know that when they send me a fresh patient, I'm not gonna fuck them up. PT + PT should be the easiest collaboration of all time. But only if we understand where the other is coming from.

So, how can the two fields collaborate to give the best patient/client care possible? How can we work together to improve their injury as best we can, while also recognizing that people can't stay in injury-prevention mode their whole life? We talk to each other and agree on a plan for care. Improvements in athleticism only come with some risk, some trial and error, some pushing when you don't want to push. Physical therapy alone isn't enough stimulus for real-life fitness. But you can't ignore it either—some things really do need that individual focus and isolation. When we work together, we cover everything, and our client gets better.

This collaboration also needs to extend into medicine. I cannot tell you the amount of truly awful fitness advice that people receive from their primary care doctors, orthopedists, and surgeons. The number of clients I've had who go to their doctor with knee pain and their doctor says, "Well, just stop running," makes me want to scream. I once had a client with long-term, very obvious, posterior tibialis tendinopathy and her primary care doctor told her she must have sprained her ankle during a workout with me. Eh?? I said there was no way that was possible, yet there she was, getting treated for an ankle sprain. I had another client who had a brain implant for her Parkinson's and I offered to talk with her doctor about safe return to exercise and she said, "Oh, he would never take your call." Oh, ok. One surgeon told my client that she didn't need a minute of physical therapy or personal training after her knee replacement, that she should let it heal on its own. What on earth. Doctors often still recommend icing and resting injuries when they occur. (FYI, resting and icing injuries has been well-debunked at this point. It's not just not helpful, it can be actively detrimental to healing. The man who invented the famous Rest/Ice/Compression/ Elevation protocol in 1978, Dr. Gabe Mirkin, revised his own work in 2015. He admitted that research supports movement and no ice, and rescinded his original RICE recommendations. Even though that was ten years ago now, plenty of doctors and physical therapists are still stuck in 1978 when it comes to icing and resting.) It goes on and on. Doctors are usually great at doctoring and very bad at personal training.

Dealing with doctors's bad fitness advice is tricky. People think you sound arrogant as hell when you argue against a doctor. I used to just be like, "That's the dumbest fucking thing I've ever heard in my life," but some clients were turned off by my assumption that I knew more about the situation than their medical provider. So I've learned how to gently wiggle my way through it instead. Now, when my client tells me their doctor told them never to squat again because it's dangerous, I'm more like, "Okay, soooooo, I hear that, and I know it's a doctor, but current practice in exercise recommends squatting as a healthy part of maintaining leg strength and general good body function. After all, without squatting, going to the bathroom might be tricky. I'd be happy to call them to ask for their advice on helping you poop while standing up. Can you give me their number?" This usually does it, and then we can get back to our regularly scheduled program. If doctors don't seek out extra fitness education, most have very little. Medical school doesn't cover it and neither does medical practice. Personally, I won't go to any kind of doctor who does not exercise themselves, because I know for a fact that they won't try to understand me or give me advice that can help me live my best. When you're dealing with a client who is following horrendous fitness advice from a medical professional, just try to publicly go along with it, and then continue doing what you know is best for your client in any way you can. But doctors: PLEASE either learn more, or trust us more. You know what would make you trust us more? Answering our fucking phone calls.

The real dream scenario is a system of collaborative care where doctors, surgeons, physical therapists, and personal trainers are all in communication about our patients/clients. We get people up close, often multiple times a week, one-on-one, for longer than anyone else. We aren't limited by insurance. We can directly influence a client's long-term physical wellbeing more than anyone else. And yes, we need more education to do our jobs well. Part of that education should come directly from the medical professionals our clients see before us. Talk to us!

I'd also like to see fitness conferences which are intended to be for doctors, trainers, and physical therapists together, rather than conferences for each profession. Part of the conference would emphasize how the three fields can better collaborate and understand each other. Why does this not exist yet?!

Finally, we need a fitness and gym industry that supports the real intentions of personal training, which is to improve people via movement. To give them the highest quality of life that they can have, at any age and ability. We don't need gyms that hire weekend-certified trainers and then require them to complete a million sessions per week just for dollars. We don't need a bunch of young jacked dudes who learned how to lift badly in the baseball locker room to be the predominant trainers on the floor of every gym. We need conferences that improve knowledge about more than high school and D1 athletes, featuring diverse panels of presenters. We need more stringent certification requirements, including general late-stage rehab, and more demanding continuing-education. And we need health professionals to respect each other's work, strengths, and limitations. I'm not so naive to think that I can change the world of medicine. But if any doctors or surgeons are reading: You're not the only one treating your person. Get as many minds on the case as it takes. Because here's what our egos love to forget: it's not about us, no matter how great we are at our jobs. It's about the person in front of us who just wants to feel better, and most people need more than one health professional in order to feel better. They deserve our collaborations. All of us are needed to complete a person's care. As my friend Ali says, every field has its brilliances, biases, and blindspots. If we have each other's backs, nothing gets missed. If we have each other's backs, we can combine our powers to get people to where they want to be. It's our duty. I'm personally ready to collaborate with each and every one of you that I can, and you should be ready to collaborate with me too.

Except Jason and Evil Josh. They can fuck off.

TL;DR:

1) Collaborative care is essential to client health. Start keeping a list of the doctors, surgeons, and physical therapists who are giving your clients good advice.

2) Instead of shitting all over people on social media, start up a conversation with them in real life. Trainers, call your clients PTs. Physical therapists, get in touch with your patient's personal trainer. Doctors, leave the fitness to the fitness professionals.

3) No one can fix everyone. Get your ego out of the picture and use your education and resources to figure out how you can get your client the best care.

4) There are a lot of assholes featured in this chapter. Don't be an asshole.

Chapter Eleven: Thoughts on the Industry

(this one goes to eleven)

Are you thirsty? Because this is the chapter where I bring you all the tea: everything from the people I hated training the most, to the influencers who make me the most crazy, to the medical practices that I hate, to the conferences that were a biggest waste of my time. (I'm so tired of hearing a hundred white dudes talk to me about hypertrophy for baseball.) Not to mention to my unending battles with lunatics who love to scream that fruit makes you fat and that a $700, sleek, rosemary-scented, olive oil vagina dock is the perfect way to promote a robust cellular environment. (Now available at GOOP!)

For every ounce of joy that I have for my job in particular, I have a nearly equal amount of horror for the industry that I work in. If you're not into reading rants, I would skip this chapter. Otherwise, join me, you gossipy hyena.

Like all jobs, there's the part of the health world which is presented to the public, and then the part of it which you only see from the inside. Unfortunately, both can be absolute trash. The elitism, the exclusion, the judgement, the emphasis on youth, the deliberate misinformation for sales, the relentless pressure to be thin enough for people to respect you as a person; these are all well-known, toxic parts of the industry I otherwise choose and love.

I blame most of the toxicity on a lack of education, cultural fatphobia, and the horrifying cultural prevalence of making things as fast as fucking possible. I despise instant health-change recommendations. Could we maybe teach the value of committing actual time to your well-being? People already understand very little about their bodies, which makes them vulnerable to all kinds of bullshit. We don't need to add five-minute workouts to the mix.

People deserve way better than what the industry gives us. We're taught—by doctors, teachers, parents, and media—that all people should *want* the same thing for their body and *do* the same thing for their body to *get* the same thing for their body. What's the thing? Striving for thinness. That's garbage. Everyone is individual and cannot be blanketed by the one driving assumption that no matter what else, all bodies should be rail thin. And yet here we are, still being trashy about it.

Body weight and shape are prevalent topics in health and fitness. This includes weight loss, weight gain, muscle size gain, body fat percentage changes, etc. Most people outside of the industry assume that helping people lose weight is my primary work, but it's not. I consider myself a weight-neutral trainer. I do not care about a client's body weight. I am there to teach everyone how to exercise safely in a body that they respect and feel love for and take care of. That's it. I don't talk about weight with any of my clients unless they talk about it with me. However, I feel a global obligation to talk about weight with everyone else, because I know that as a health professional, I can make a positive difference here.

Fat bias is in your life and in your history. Start your training career by trying to unlearn it. You can absolutely be a trainer who specializes in helping people with weight loss, but you HAVE to decenter fatphobia in order to do it. I didn't do this for years as a trainer because the cultural bias is so deeply ingrained I didn't even know it was there. The history is thicc, and not in a good way. But you can do it long before I (and many others) managed to, by recognizing some of that history now.

We blew into the 1950's with "fat bad" and "thin good" and haven't looked back since. This is still the predominant medical take, even though good health is never a single-issue assessment to make. There are a thousand things that could be deviating in a body, and it is a health provider's responsibility to look at all of them, gain an understanding of the situation, and only then make recommendations. To see a fat person with entirely healthy parameters and say, "You need to lose weight," is short-sighted and unfair. Even worse if they never bother to ask about their lifestyle habits, assuming instead that they don't have any good ones. I have plenty of fat friends and family, with no health concerns, whose doctors told them to lose weight without ever even asking if they eat vegetables, exercise, or manage stress. That's for shit. You can be better than many doctors simply by directing all your clients on the best way to incorporate healthy habits rather than talking about the scale.

In personal training, don't let it be enough for someone to tell you they just want to lose pounds. If they're coming to see you about their weight, try to get at why they want to lose weight and what they think weight loss will do for them. For some, it's as simple as not feeling good in their body. I've had many clients drop twenty to forty pounds, keep it off, and feel much better. Great. For others, the weight isn't actually their problem, they've just been told it is by a fatphobic diet culture that pins every unhappiness on body size. They're hoping your exercise will finally be the change they need. And it can be! But not in the way they think. Helping them to de-center the weight-loss part and center the habit-change part is critical.

Weight is one aspect of a human body, but it's not the only aspect. No responsible cardiologist would see that someone has high blood pressure with otherwise healthy parameters and immediately say, "You need to have a bypass." That cardiologist would check out the heart's function, the tissue quality, the surrounding blood vessels, the person's lifestyle, etc, before recommending a course of action. You need to do the same thing with your clients. Don't assume a client wants to lose weight; don't decide for them that they need to. Not all fat people are struggling or interested in changing sizes. If someone tells you that they do want to lose weight, help them explore why. (In general, exploring why a client wants to achieve anything is a critical trainer skill. Remember, you're part therapist.) One of the most important things a personal trainer can do to help other people is work on busting the umbrella idea of "fat bad" and "thin good."

Of course, there are tons of studies suggesting that excess weight combined with poor lifestyle habits can cause major health problems. No one is arguing with that. But this is really important: researchers are still not sure if it's the weight or the habits. Either way, we know absolutely that the obsession and fixation on reducing scale numbers, instead of obsessing and fixating on improving the poor lifestyle habits, is totally backwards. Teaching people to improve their lifestyle habits because it will make them healthier—independently of whether it changes their weight or not—is the way. It creates a compassionate, realistic, measurable, and sustainable plan that can be successfully implemented over time without the shame, humiliation, and feelings of failure that come with constant dieting and weight anguish. Improving nutrition, adding regular exercise, getting better sleep, and managing stress makes fat people healthier. Period. And here's the bias part: *This exact same thing is true for thin people. It's just that we all think it's only fat people who need to change everything they're doing and become healthier.*

Every single person except for Chris Traeger from Parks and Rec has some unhealthy habits. (And his fanaticism, while hilarious, was in itself extremely unhealthy.) But we only hate fat people for having those habits. If a thin person says, "I don't have time to exercise," most people would nod their heads in understanding. If a fat person says it, people hear it as, "I'm lazy," "I have no willpower," or "I'm a slob." They'll tell the person to find time, and eat less while they're at it. This is not altruistic concern for someone else's health, as the internet commenters always say. This is fat bias and it is devastating. If you showed a group of a people a picture of me eating a donut, they'd wonder what they were supposed to notice in the picture. No one cares when I eat a donut. But if you showed a group of people a fat person eating a donut, most of them would say (or think), "They shouldn't be eating that." The donut has the same amount of calories no matter who is eating it, but our standards for who is healthy and who deserves to eat are not equal.

Because of this fat prejudice, the nuance for obesity treatment has never moved past "fat bad" and "thin good." We can't seem to look beyond the number on the scale no matter how many people call for more nuance. Many people more qualified than I have argued that the emotional damage caused by our intense, very public, societal fatphobia is more damaging to people than the physical excess weight on their frame. Depression and anxiety rates among bigger people are massive and can last for decades or lifetimes. It is reasonable to suggest that treating the mood disorders caused by cultural norms, properly teaching healthy lifestyle habits rather than scale-number focus, and working to reduce social fatphobia for the next generation, would have a far more positive and lasting effect on public health than screaming for everyone to lose weight. Certainly better than shame, black-and-white statements, and restrictive diets, all of which harm everybody.

Our society, medicine, and the fitness industry have done irreparable damage to countless people. One of the most common things I've read from fat authors and educators is that fat people feel invisible unless they lose weight. Can you take a second to hear that? Can you try to imagine how devastating it would be to realize that people will only see you as a human if you get thinner? Not anything about your behavior or personality. Only human if you're thin. Fat people have a harder time getting jobs, getting adequate medical care, and let's not forget that anti-fat bias can actually drive weight gain. You, as a weight-neutral trainer, even though you are just one person, can be a powerful voice to combat all of that judgment. You can be one loud voice in the opposition. You're a health expert seeing them and telling them they're doing alright as they are. That cannot be overvalued in today's cultural climate.

That toxic judgy cultural climate doesn't quit at just food or fat, either. We judge other people for EVERYTHING. For sleep and exercise and supplements and sunscreen and childbearing and child rearing and driving skills and doing too many or not enough health screens and having the wrong insurance and taking the wrong vitamins and staring at phones and listening to music too loud and and and and and and. Surf the comments on any health-related social media post and feel depressed forever. Most of us are deeply undereducated but full of angry ideas about what other people are doing wrong for their health. It's one of the worst parts of the industry, and it's where health professionals can make the biggest difference to patients, clients, and even the people reading and being brainwashed by those same internet comments.

Education and broad-mindedness is the combat line for health professionals. We need to learn as much as we can, be open to new ideas that contradict our old ideas, and talk with other health professionals, especially the ones whose work is not like our own. We need to question if what we've been taught might not have been correct, even if it came from a reputable source. If we're really going to make a difference to our clients, then we need to pay better attention to them as individuals. We need to meet people where they are instead of meeting them at some arbitrary standard. Show them how to care for themselves in the ways in which they struggle the most, which is almost always the big concepts of health: eat a ton of plants and protein; move every day, sleep long and deep, talk about your feelings, see sunlight. Being the guide who brings one of these concepts to people is a deeply gratifying part of the job. Because we've all seen a stratospheric level of health bullshit in our lives already and no one wants more.

The problem? Bullshit sells.

Health education has been a profitable shitshow in the United States for a hundred years. Look at the diet advice our parents had to grow up with. The smoking diet (created by the tobacco industry); the sugar-based diet (created by the sugar industry); the tuna diet (created by the tuna industry); the milk diet (created by the dairy industry, are you starting to see a theme?); the pineapple diet (simply pictures of hot women next to pieces of pineapple, kind of iconic tbh); intentional tapeworms (jesus fucking christ); weight loss pills (still relevant and depressing in 2024); apple cider vinegar, Mrs. Dash and lemon juice; even the famous food pyramid—which every child my age had to memorize—has long been accused of being under the control of various food and agriculture industries to make their particular section more prominent.

The debates rage on today: Atkins, intermittent fasting, gluten sensitivity, nutritional timing, Mediterranean, intuitive eating, plant-based plates, the Whole 30, etc. No one has enough time in their life to give every type of plan a go. That's why nutrition education for all of us, starting with medical doctors, needs to be way better. People need guidance from the providers who know them best. The new mom doesn't need intermittent fasting—she barely has time to pee. She finally gets an opportunity to eat and you're gonna tell her it's outside her timing window? Fuck no. Tell her to stockpile as much protein as she can, eat a ton of berries, greens, and grains, and stop counting calories to lose baby weight. Childbirth is traumatic AND she's feeding two people. It's not the time for the fucking Atkins diet.

We could be doing so much better for people here. (Remember, trainers aren't qualified to give nutrition plans. But doctors sure should be.)

Interestingly, for as bad as the nutritional content was in the last century, a lot of the old-school fitness advice was quite good. Jog. Lift free weights. Gym class calisthenics. Aerobics. Gymnastics. Martial arts. Yoga. Even the biggest fitness trends have been pretty good. Mock Jazzercise if you must, but it got a ton of people, especially women, moving often. Kettlebells, TaeBo, Spinning, Zumba. Step Aerobics. All fantastic for general fitness.

Unfortunately for general fitness, the internet was invented.

Previously, there were just a few voices preaching about fitness. Jane Fonda, Richard Simmons, Jack Lalanne, Billy Blanks. All GOATs. Now? A hellscape of fitfluencers and bloggers with bad advice covered by hot bodies. As Olivia Rodrigo says, it's brutal out there. Of course there is excellent fitness information on the web, but it isn't always easy to find. And a beginner would not be able to distinguish bad advice from good advice just by reading social feeds. Number of followers ain't it. Quantity of posting ain't it. Even advanced degrees ain't always it (there are some real fucking jackasses pimping their PhD's alongside their clowning shitposts). Plus, we social media consumers have an attention problem, which makes it harder for everyone.

What captures our attention on the internet is, unfortunately, not great educational content. What captures our attention is beauty, video-making skills, and humor. People love to laugh more than anything. One memorable line in a viral video can be all it takes for people to adopt that opinion, no matter how wrong it might be. You remember the line from the movie *Sideways*? About how he's not drinking fucking merlot? That one line damaged the merlot industry for years, because people who knew nothing about wine suddenly knew that they should drink anything but merlot. When people don't have any education on a topic, one funny line can form a wrong opinion fast. This happens in fitness posts all the time. But where bad wine information isn't going to affect your life, bad fitness information really, really can.

The internet is a pit of people looking to promote themselves and disguise it as helping you. It's a never-ending game for attention. If you're trying to get your online personal training/programming going, good for you, but don't act like you're playing a different game than everyone else. Even for the best-intentioned people, it can't be any other way. The algorithms force it. The game consists of: hot body pics; the ability to do impressive shit; youth/thinness/beauty; and spouting aggressive, often negative opinions, because people arguing with you in the comment section is great for engagement and we all know it. Fitness social media has created an entire world where in order to promote your own version of healthy exercise, you have to shit all over something else in order to make your point. It's not enough to say what you are. You have to say what you are not, and the more controversially you say it, the more your posts get shown to people.

I hate-follow a bunch of people and companies on IG. Why? I'm not sure. My hate-follow only gives them another follower. But I can't help it. I love a trainwreck. I love the people who take a reasonable fitness concept and transform it into a giant steaming dump on the floor. If you produce poop and sell poop, that's fine. You're honest about the poop. But if you produce poop and call it diamonds, that sucks. Because the average user doesn't know any better. They'll see a slick video of a jacked body and flashy graphics promising unscientific pain relief and be sucked in like a moth to a porch light. Even worse, the caption says something like this:

Hey! You! Stop scrolling! Are you stretching your quads before you run, you cunt? Who told you to do that? Someone at yoga?! Gross. Static stretching will lengthen your tissues and ligaments uncontrollably until you get BACK PAIN and SCIATICA. Also KNEE PAIN and probably OTHER PAIN. Does your shoulder hurt? EXACTLY. Can you say instability?? And you're doing that every day?! YIKES. You're stuck in a FEEDBACK LOOP of HORMONES and CHEMICALS.

Don't make us say it again: STATIC STRETCHING WILL KILL YOU.

Unless...it's OUR static stretching!!!! It's a ten week program, only $900, and it will FIX YOU. How? Well, you'll find out after you buy it, won't you! Remember, kids, yoga kills.

Sounds scary, right? It's poop, but it looks shiny to the outsider. Sooo many people will read this trash and think, *Holy shit, I fucked up my whole body just by stretching? I had no idea.* Meanwhile Billy Madison Fitness Patterns didn't actually make a single coherent point. Every reader is dumber for having read that caption, and may God have mercy on their soul. (Trainer Tip Side Note #1: People ask about stretching all the time, so let's just clear the air while we're here. Stretching is fine. It may or may not get you the given result you're looking for [it won't prevent injuries, for example], but it's fine. If you could permanently deform your body's tissues just by stretching for a few seconds, we'd be fucked every time we stepped over a high fence, reached across the dining room table, or bent down to pick something up off the floor. We'd stumble around like those floaty guys outside of car dealerships, doomed to an eternity of increasingly flaccid collapse.)

(Increasingly Flaccid Collapse is going to be the name of my sex memoir from college.)

Social media is all about being vague while pretending to be super specific. You're trying to write a post about one specific topic but make it sound like it applies to everyone. That's impossible, but it doesn't stop people from trying. That's how you end up with fear-mongering captions like the one above. Specificity doesn't sell, so people opt for vague and scary. Don't fall for this. Vagueness is a guarantee that someone doesn't know what they're talking about. If an account never gives specifics, then they don't have any specifics to give. Go somewhere else for information.

But my biggest gripe about social media fitness (and social media in general) is not my hate-follows. It's that social media puts every single user on the same level of expertise. It's literally designed to be an equalizer: everyone's opinion can be heard at equal volume. That's the whole point of social media: volume equality. Social media is designed to make everyone feel like the entire world can, will, and wants to hear them.

The problem is that not all of those billions of opinions are equally knowledgable, valid, or safe. People are not equally educated on any given topic. But the nature of the platform says we are, and it also says that the way to distinguish the extra good ones is by how many followers they have. So some jackass with a million followers and a six-pack can talk about how your butt turns off and his $1200 program will fix it and people will believe him. (Trainer Tip Side Note #2: your butt does not turn off. It can become deregulated by pain, habits, and neurological pattern changes. But it does not turn off.)

So with everyone being presented as a potential expert, how can you distinguish useful information on social media from not-useful information? First, ask your knowledgable friends. Word-of-mouth from experts is the best way. Ask your other trainer friends who they follow and support. Testimonials are also useful. Head into the comment section (beware, lol). Is it full of skeptics? Full of supporters? All of my hate-follows have tons of skeptics in the comments and for good reason: they post inaccurate or unproven or dangerous information. People call them out for it. You can also cross-check the information they're giving. A quick surfing of Google will often disprove wild claims. But more than anything, take EVERYTHING on social media with a grain of salt, even stuff from trustworthy people. There is little room for specificity, nuance, or detail in any post. People are forced to summarize complex topics in just a few sentences, and that summary gets sold and distributed as iron-clad fact. Say it with me: social media is not the best place to get health information of any kind. Go ahead. Say it. Social / media / is / not / the / best/ place / to / get / health / information / of / any / kind.

I'd tell you to just go out and find someone in person, but that's not a cinch either. The world is full of wellness terrorists, on social media and well beyond it. Too many people who want to throw napalm on our insecurities, our phobias, and our fear of aging, in order to sell us something expensive to cure it. Bonus points for using words that sound healthy: natural, authentic, organic, functional, enhancer, recovery, performance, etc. I mean, buy whatever you want, yay capitalism, but a $90 water bottle doesn't hold water better than a $10 water bottle. It's just that someone told you it did—likely by suggesting it would make you fitter, younger, or thinner—and you believed them.

A majority of things for sale in the United States is tied to our health in some way or another, especially for women. Like at large clothing retailers, where they put signs all around the women's clothing sections like *Smooth and sleek* to describe tank tops and *Firming and tightening* to describe leggings. It's all code for *These clothes will make you look thinner,* which, if you were wondering, doesn't happen in the men's section. Their signs say really wild things like *Shirts* and *Pants.* And, of course, in the shampoo and conditioner aisle of any drug store in

America, you'll find a hundred bottles ready to cure women. *For the shabby, weak, fragile, dry, brittle, and gross rat nests on top of your itchy, flaky, toxic, disgusting head.*

The men's bottles? *For hair.*

This obsession with selling youth, vibrance, and shininess is maybe most prevalent in the fitness industry, because that's still what sells health and fitness better than anything else. Equinox has never made an advertisement with someone over size two / age twenty-five, and also leans HEAVILY into the *You will get laid as part of your membership* side of things. Which, like, okay, but I personally don't need a side of orgy with my battle ropes.

One large company used to put insane things on their social media, including one graphic where an obese statue was chiseling himself into a skinny statue, alongside a caption saying it was finally time to become a better person. Yikes. They also posted a Valentine's Day post which showed a young woman lifting a weight with her trainer looming closely over her, with ad copy that said, *The unexpected results of weightlifting.* It still gives me the heebie jeebies. What's the unexpected result? Men getting in your personal space, your trainer inappropriately asking you out, or sexual assault? Who's to know? I emailed the company to ask, but strangely, they didn't answer.

Interestingly, both Planet Fitness and Crossfit (two much-maligned brands in the fitness world) do a much better job. Their marketing tends to represent the work of fitness, rather than the physical outcomes of fitness. I love this, even though I don't love either of their overall marketing strategies. (Planet Fitness, the judgement-free zone with an entire massive ad campaign about the people who are not allowed to be in their clubs. And Crossfit, where the message is that above all else, your workouts should leave you weeping in a corner. But I'll credit Crossfit for improving their image a whole lot from the days of Uncle Rhabdo and Pukey the Clown.) Both of their ads still largely feature young and thin people but not exclusively. It's something.

Unfortunately, fitness marketers in general know what they're doing. They know that young, thin bodies still sell the best, and few companies want to give up that image if it means they won't sell as many gym memberships. It's the part of the industry that makes me the saddest, because what we trainers see in real life isn't anything like these brazen, sweaty, hardbody ad campaigns. We see everyday people busting their asses to get a decent lunge; slow, tedious mobility work to help people climb the stairs to their house; everybody struggling through cardio because in spite of what marketers want you to think, cardio is hardio for everyone, not just fat people.

More people would work out if we could get the industry to stop glorifying a body type and start glorifying working your ass off because it's great for living longer with fewer problems. How many orgies do I have to attend to get Equinox to do some posts about synovial fluid or combatting ligamentous changes with age? Who does a girl have to screw around here to get some social media posts about kidneys and colons? And how do we get two billion Instagram users to care about videos of a sixty-year old woman doing three slow pushups on a bench, in the way that they care about videos of a twenty-year old guy doing backflips with a barbell?

Well, some accounts and companies are trying, and I applaud them because it's slow-going. It's easy to sell *Come here and become hot,* or *Come here and cure your pain.* It's not easy to sell *It depends.* Constantly writing "it depends" in response to general fitness questions is a great way to lose viewers. People don't want it. They want answers. They want instant fixes. They want those god-awful "POV" videos where someone shows a random exercise and then claims that it will make all your back pain go away.

Guys, those videos suck ass. Imagine if you were having problems learning French. And someone online goes, *POV: You're struggling with French but then you learn this one verb and all your problems go away.* Stupid, right? Learning one verb will never teach you an entire language, just like learning one exercise will never teach you how to care for your body. These videos only sound like they makes sense because people are undereducated about how their bodies work. Plus, we all want a magic solution. Modern western medicine has deeply ingrained in us that when there is a problem, there is a) a specific cause and b) a specific solution. That is rarely the case, especially with musculoskeletal stuff.

There's a reason you don't see doctors on Instagram saying, *POV: You've got a bellyache but then you have this one surgery and it goes away.* As personal trainers, we're supposed to take our clients' health as seriously as doctors take their patients' health. We're supposed to be helping individual people move better, not just batting their back pain around for likes and subscriptions. This is one reason why personal trainers are regularly mocked by physical therapists, doctors, surgeons, etc, for being useless, dumb, and often dangerous. Because all they see is our awful POV videos and I can't blame them. There are so many great personal trainers who can't get traction online because they're not willing to compromise their beliefs for the algorithm. So these assclowns who are perfectly willing to post flaming garbage in the name of internet clout destroy all of our reputations and the industry suffers.

The personal trainer reputation is grim, on and off social media. Aside from removal of the assclowns, we need three other things to improve the world of personal training: more education for trainers, higher standards of job performance, and trainers with more diverse life experience. The combination is key. Stringent trainer education, alongside diligent supervisors who ensure trainer performance, plus the life experience of people who discovered fitness after college, who are older, who are female, who are of color, who are disabled, is the linchpin to a better industry. Otherwise we just have a bunch of young, able-bodied men throwing random high school hypertrophy techniques at a post-menopausal woman who's never played a sport in her life. It rarely works. That woman doesn't feel seen, so she gets spooked and leaves. Meanwhile the trainer learns that older women are spookable and liable to leave. They don't try as hard next time. No one improves. The industry needs growth from the inside in order to reach and keep people from the outside.

Except, the industry isn't interested in growth. Take continuing education, for example. Continuing education in the field is currently self-taught and minimally tracked. I've never been required to demonstrate or improve my education as a trainer, other than the minimums for recertification. (This minimum can be covered by attending two conferences in three years. You don't need to demonstrate any actual learning at the conferences, just that you went to them.) Job performance is rarely, if ever, evaluated. Most chain gyms don't care about the *quality* of their trainers' work, they care about the *quantity* of it. If a bad trainer is doing 150 bad sessions a month, their boss is still gonna be thrilled. I've never had a boss sit me down and ask me the ways in which I've been working to improve my skill set and client care.

Most gyms also don't care about the diversity of their training staff. Trainers typically diverge by gender in their specialities. Women tend to dominate general health and fitness, including teaching group exercise classes. Men tend to dominate strength and conditioning. Men rarely teach the "girly" classes. Women are not seen as equally capable of coaching strength. (This is well-documented, even for very young kids, and especially boys.) Just improving the gender diversity of these two basic fitness positions would be huge. But we need gyms to make efforts for their racial diversity too. People of color face multiple barriers in the industry, which is overwhelmingly white in its leadership. Feminine men, women, trainers with disabilities, and trainers of color are not generally encouraged to take leadership positions in health and fitness. So the heads of the industry, the ones presenting at the biggest conferences and the ones regularly being featured in the media, are nearly always masculine white men. And the conferences usually suck.

All but one fitness conference I've ever been to featured 90% to 100% masculine white men as the presenters and keynote speakers. This isn't an indictment of masculine white men so much as an indictment of companies only asking masculine white men to present. Last year's summit for one of the biggest conference companies (let's call them SuperDuper Fitness), a highly-respected conference in the field, had twenty-six men, three women, one speaker of color. Which is hardly better than when I attended the conference in 2018, which had eleven men, one woman, one speaker of color. When I wrote an email at the time to ask why they weren't doing better at this, they let me know that their attendees prefer to see white men:

When we look for presenters to speak at our conferences we do not look at race, color or gender to make our selection. We are not trying to fill a quota. What we are looking for are the best presenters in the industry. We get this list from evaluations that we do regularly as well as hundreds of people emailing us each year as to who they want to listen to.

- SuperDuper Fitness, January 10, 2018

My reply:

SuperDuper Fitness is one of the most impressive names in fitness, with a wide audience and very public view. One of the ways that an industry conveys its values is in who it decides should be the face of its biggest organizations. In a large-scale presentation of eight different seminars, all of which will be led by white men, SuperDuper Fitness conveys that it most values white men's opinions. (And, in fact, you suggest similar by implying the only reason to invite women and minorities would be to fill quotas.) The science of fitness is diverse, and deserves to be represented that way.

Crickets.

I've also had a multi-year argument with the NSCA, my own certifying body, about their lack of conference speaker diversity. When I called to talk with them about it (and props to them for having multiple calls and meetings with me on this issue), they also told me that they ask their membership who they want to hear as speakers, and their membership tends to vote for men. They also told me in 2018 that their membership divide was 80% men, 20% women and in spite of many efforts, had never been able to move the needle on that stat. (Last I heard, they are now 70/30.) Can't move the needle? I can't speak for how people of color in the industry feel, but it's not hard to make the connection that when women only see male speakers in the field, discussing topics that apply primarily to male athletes, they lose interest in the field. It's not rocket science. The field of strength and conditioning simply wasn't, and still isn't, made for us. I was happy, however, to see that this year's NSCA conference features an improved speaker diversity, with a much more diverse array of topics. A good start.

Perhaps unsurprisingly, the worst conference I've ever been to was the SuperDuper Fitness Speaker Conference. It's a conference specifically designed to help get people prepared for lecturing in fitness, something I've always wanted to do. The world of lecturing is notoriously tough to break into. No one wants to trust you without knowing you've spoken somewhere else and you didn't fuck it up. So good luck getting anyone to book you with no experience. It's brutal, which is exactly why (I thought) this conference exists.

This conference was intended to help improve our pitching skills, presentation skills, give feedback/workshopping to others, and improve our network. The guy running it (I'll call him Brian) is one of the biggest names in the industry, who, as he told us multiple times, makes a fortune giving hundreds of talks a year. I was really excited for this course. Finally, a place where I could get a leg in the door, both in terms of help with pitching topics and getting some inside connections in the industry.

As the weekend approached, I emailed to ask how many, what length, and what types of talks we should prepare in advance. They said, "None. You'll work on it when you're there." A red flag, but I ignored it.

I shouldn't have.

For starters, I was the only woman in the class of about twenty-two people. That alone sets me on edge, but I tried to see it as an opportunity to stand up for the very thing I've been fighting for: to prove that women know what they're talking about when it comes to strength and conditioning. At this conference, I could demonstrate that my knowledge was every bit as good as those twenty-one men. Well, Brian didn't care about anyone's knowledge except Brian's.

After introductions, the very first thing we did was look at a slide of a woman lifting weights. Brian asked us what we thought about the picture. As a group, we said things like, "She looks like she's enjoying herself," and "She seems to know what she's doing in the gym." After we made about ten comments, Brian looked at all of us perplexed. He finally said, "Hm. Ok. Well, the first thing that most people notice is that she's fat."

The room went silent. He went on to explain that, just like in personal training, first impressions of appearance make all the difference when it comes to an audience respecting a speaker. I think everyone in the room was deeply uncomfortable. We were only twenty minutes in, and I already felt dread for the rest of the weekend.

After sufficiently fat-shaming the woman in his slide (and, it won't surprise you to know, she had a perfectly average body type), we went to the gym across the hall. Time to start improving our own appearances. Everyone took turns walking down the turf floor, as if we were walking across a stage to begin our presentation. I swear to god. We practiced walking. He let me know that I was walking too much like a woman, with my hips swinging side-to-side and my feet criss-crossing each other. (He gave a cartoonish demo to be sure we all understood what he was saying.) He taught me to walk with my feet wide, in order to give a more commanding presence when I step on stage. When I was hobbling down the turf floor like a cowboy who shit his pants, he nodded approval. In an unrelated story, it cost $1,650 to attend this course.

After walking time, Brian went through and critiqued the appearance of most people in the class. He told all the men with beards and long hair to shave and get a haircut—by the next day. He told me to wear more colors and makeup. He instructed everyone to dress up for the next day of our conference, and cautioned that the men who did not shave would not receive high marks. (High marks in what? you might ask. The answer is high marks in power dynamics from a wimpy man who wants to control people.)

Eventually, we practiced speaking...by standing up one time, cold turkey, in the front of the room, and ad-libbing a presentation about fitness for five minutes. No preparation, no practice, nothing written, and with no specific topic suggestion. He took great joy in letting all of us know that we sucked at it. But we wouldn't suck by the end of the weekend! Uh. What? Of course we sucked. Please go stand up right now and speak for five minutes straight about anything. Let me know if it's conference-ready. For fuck's sake.

At this point I was like, oh, this is the game? We intentionally don't prepare anything, then we give that same five-minute talk all weekend long so by the end it looks like he's molded us into perfect speakers with a conference-ready lecture in hand?

Turns out I was still giving way too much credit.

On day two, we all returned, dressed up. Many of the men had shaved, but not all of them, and Brian let them know he was displeased. I respected the hell out of those guys. Over morning coffee, Brian had a couple of the freshly-shaven guys stand up in place, so we could see them. "Better?" he asked the room. We all murmured assent. I know I wasn't the only one who hated this.

And me? I didn't just stand up in place. Brian asked me to come to the front of the room. (Remember, I'm the only woman there.) I shyly went up in my teal shirt, black blazer, black pants, heels, and makeup. I felt like meat for sale, standing in front of twenty-one men while Brian said, "How does she look? Scale of 1-10." I looked at him, panicked, and then immediately identified every emergency exit in the room so I could quickly launch myself into the sun.

"Eight," someone offered.

"Seven?" another person wondered.

I tried to joke, like any zoo animal would. "Seven?????????????" I said, cracking an emotionless smile.

"Seven is good. I agree. Much better. You can sit down," Brian said. I crawled back to my seat.

I figured out quickly that Brian's favorite game was Ask Me Questions. This is something that blowhards do when they're too lazy to prepare any kind of lesson plan. They assume that the room is dying to know their every thought and secret, so they just sit up there on their throne asking for people's questions. He started this early on Day Two, with the guise of the PowerPoint slides still up on the projector behind him. On Day Three? Didn't even bother with slides. He just sat on the table at the front of the room, told us he wouldn't be teaching anything else, and that we would just do questions for the day. The day! Nine hours! Of questions!

The promo for the specific weekend I went to, which is still online, says that you can learn to be a great speaker with intensive practice. Sounds pretty good, yes? Even if the theme of the weekend was being douchy and out of touch, at least we got intensive speaking practice in, yeah?

Nope.

I spoke two times that weekend, for five minutes each.

The conference was 8am to 5pm, three days in a row. We were together for twenty-seven hours in a conference about intensively improving one's speaking skills and I spoke in front of the room for ten total minutes. I already told you about the first time: cold-turkey, no prep. I spoke the second time on Day Two. There had not been any work done on my presentation between attempt one and attempt two. Just time passing. Brian's critique on this round was unique and interesting and has never been given by a man to a woman before: he told me I needed to smile more and that I spoke in a monotonous voice. If I'd known he was looking for me to radiate happiness the whole time, I would have just made my presentation about how to tune out soggy, ignorant men when they're on tiny-dick-waving power trips. My voice would have been positively lilting!

On the morning of Day Three, Brian said he didn't have any more information to share. As far as I remember, no one did any presenting on Day Three. If they did, it certainly wasn't all of us. I don't remember how we spent the day other than asking Brian questions, but I did not speak again at the speaking conference. While writing this chapter, I reached out to many of my classmates to double-check my memory. All but one confirmed that they spoke either two or three times all weekend. One guy said, "Can you believe I flew across the country for that conference? Ouch."

The ickiest part was—and hold onto your hats here because you're gonna be shocked—Brian's rampant sexism. There were several instances, but the worst one was when Brian decided to tell a story about being at the airport. I'll write the story as I remember it here:

I was in the airport bathroom and as I walked in, I noticed two pairs of feet under the stall. [He raised his eyebrows up and down salaciously at the room.] *I used the bathroom but when I came out, they were gone. However, I noticed a woman's scarf in the stall where they'd been. Now, I had seen their shoes, so I took the scarf and started wandering the nearby terminals, looking for her shoes. And then I saw them! I went straight up to her, leaned over, and said, 'You forgot this in the bathroom.'"* [Eyebrows again, delighted with himself.]

First of all, why was this story being told? The same reason bananas are blue. No one knows. I suspect it was a male crowd pleaser twenty years ago. Some of the dudes in the room politely laughed. But me? I was too stunned to do anything, because when Brian was getting to the punchline of looking for the shoes of the woman who was fucking in a bathroom stall, he was standing in front of me, looking under my desk at my feet, then standing up, leaning over me, and handing me an imaginary scarf, looking me in the eyes to say, "You forgot this in the bathroom," while the men around me politely laughed.

I instantly felt like twenty-two men, including my instructor, were imagining me having sex in an airport bathroom stall. I wanted to die. No one said a single thing and I just sat there, frozen, until the class moved on.

I spent all night at home thinking about this. I wanted to let Brian know how bad it made me feel, but I knew that it would wreck the chance that he would recommend me for anything. All women can identify the kind of man who will shut her down at a moment's notice and never look back, and Brian was definitely one of those. I tossed it around in my mind for hours, the idea of standing up for myself because it was the right thing to do vs. silently accepting it in favor of what I hoped would be given to me at the end. A classic decision that many underrepresented people must make in their respective industries.

The decision wasn't made until I walked in at eight the next morning and got instantly angry when I saw him. Fuck the career. I waited until we were on lunch break and then shyly went up to him when he was by himself. The instant he knew what the subject was, his face hardened. My heart fell. When I stopped talking, he said nothing. We stared at each other.

I lost my confidence and started to backtrack a bit. I stopped talking again when I saw his face turning red with anger.

"I have absolutely no idea what you're talking about, but sorry I guess," he said sarcastically, as he stood up and walked out of the room.

Five more hours of conference and he did not even look at me again. At the end, he asked people to come up to him and he would try to give them some parting gifts: people who spoke on the same subjects as them; contacts; advice for next steps. Amazingly, he gave me several ideas which he thought might help me.

No, I'm just kidding! He waved me away like a fly and cheerfully addressed the man standing behind me in line. I tried to stand there defiantly, but it was no use. The guy behind me stepped in front of me and I was out.

$1,650, ten minutes of improv speaking, and a blacklist. What a weekend. I sat in my car and cried for a while before driving home.

Women are still ignored and disrespected in the field of strength and conditioning. During our speaking school, Brian had said, "It's not easy to break into the field, and it's a whole lot harder for women. I'm sorry but that's just how it is." Gee, I wonder why. And the internet exacerbates it. An influencer whose content I very much like once posted a list of S&C experts that he recommended for follows. There wasn't a single woman on the list of fifteen or so. Someone else in the comments asked for some female recs and he said, verbatim, "I can't think of any women I'd recommend in S&C, but if I find any, I'll post them." This comment has haunted me for years now. Not just because he said it, but because so many of his followers would *see* that he said it. Every one of those followers learned from a trusted source that there aren't any women worth recommending in S&C.

A man in the gym once told me that we had to stop training because he doesn't like taking orders from a woman.

Another man, when I offered to spot him, said, no offense, but he just doesn't want bench pressing advice from a woman.

We have clients who want us to wear skirts when we train, or sports bras when we teach classes.

Another short-lived client of mine told me that it made him uncomfortable that I had any other men as clients. He wanted to have me for himself.

Nearly 100% of the S&C coaches in collegiate and professional sports are men, although there are now a couple women in the space. And while my personal male clients always make me feel like a valued equal, there's no question that the greater world of S&C always leaves me feeling left out. My public opinion never holds as much weight as a man's public opinion on the same topic. My training concerns and my female clients' training concerns are never treated as vitally as men's training concerns, and often not treated at all.

I hadn't realized how deep that (lack of) treatment ran until I attended a conference in 2019 called The Female Athlete Conference (hosted by Boston Children's Hospital). 80% of the speakers were female, and 100% of the talks were about issues specific to women's athletics. The difference was so jarring I almost couldn't believe it. I've attended more than fifty strength and conditioning conferences and lectures. All those years of listening carefully to speed training for football players and hip impingement concerns for hockey players and now I was suddenly hearing about progesterone and periods, the rampant rate of ACL tears in girl's soccer, and how to teach female athletes about handling their anger. (This would be a great one for men too, of course. Male-focused conferences almost never address any mental concerns.) It was revolutionary.

The solution is laughably easy. Put women at the front of the room. Put topics relevant to women at the front of the room. Discuss how exercise recommendations affect men and women differently, and make a point of the times when men and women are *not* affected differently. Read and publish research on female athletes. The number of times I've been to a conference where someone asks about the impact on women and the speaker says, "Unfortunately, they rarely do studies on women, so this only applies to men," I'm going to lose my mind. And we also need to encourage men to learn about the girls and women they train. Everything above will only even the playing field if men actually attend.

The FAC was phenomenal; the best I've ever been to. And you know how many men attended in 2019? I counted ten. The prevalence of something in fitness being "for girls" and therefore not relevant to men is still super strong.

So are all of the industry leaders assholes? It kind of sounds like it from this chapter, Mia, don't you think?

The short answer is of course not and of course yes. I genuinely believe that most people are doing the best they can with what they've got. But could industry leaders be working harder to be more inclusive? God yes. I'd love to see a mainstream fitness conference offering leadership on the latest research on trans people in sport; on giving male trainers tools to connect with their female clients about periods and pelvic floor health; on considerations for strength-training a wheelchair athlete; on modifying popular exercises for bigger bodies; on the psychology of teaching beginner female lifters. (This is one of the biggest obstacles I face in my job—women often don't know how strong they are or can become, because they are deeply hindered by social constraints.) Give us some fucking recommendations for pre-and post-natal women!!! It's kind of common!!!

Everyone could be doing better in seeking out diversity in every aspect of the field. Especially in conference speaking, where voices get amplified in ways that have major career implications. SuperDuper Fitness told me that they simply hired the speakers that their membership wanted to hear. But this doesn't work. At all. When you ask a group of uninformed people which conference speakers they would like to hear next year, they will always just choose the four names they've heard of. (This is the same psychology behind putting political lawn signs and bumper stickers everywhere. We trust the names we see repeatedly.) So those same four (white men) get selected over and over and over because we keep seeing their names over and over and over.

They become the industry leaders. They receive the most prestigious coaching jobs, speaking assignments, and consulting gigs.

Representation matters in every industry, but especially in health and fitness. The world of fitness is incredibly diverse, simply based on the fact that all humans need to exercise. We need a wide variety of trainers and industry voices who represent the scale of the human race. And we also need the trainers who do fit the classic athlete demographics to be able to train those who do not. Being able to connect with a wide variety of clients is a key to success in this field. Every client deserves a trainer who has the tools to see them for who they are and listen to what they need. Our gender, race, religion, disabilities, upbringing, age, hormones, limitations, diseases, and family situations are all critical parts of who we are and how we operate in the world. How we operate in the world nearly always indicates how we operate in the gym. So if you want to help someone make changes to how they operate in the gym (and that's why 99% of people will come see you), then you'll first need to understand how they operate in the world. This is much easier to do if you have been resourced in advance by diverse industry leaders sharing their own lived experiences.

Do you see how this works? You can't just ask a random group of conference attendees who they would like to hear and then go with it. They don't have informed opinions. It is the conference organizers who must do the research, extend invites to unknown voices who are doing great things (they're really not that hard to find), and work with them to produce meaningful, diverse lectures for those conferences. We need to be shown who the best leaders are, and a group of leaders with identical demographics can never be considered the best. Leadership leads all, not some.

One last note on the industry: if you're taking education matters into your own hands and sourcing your own information instead of waiting around for the big names in fitness to do it for you, good move! There are plenty of great influencers online selling great programs. How to find them? My rules of thumb are these:

• If someone says that their program is the only one on Planet Earth that works, run away.

• If someone promises that you will quickly earn large amounts of money as a result of buying their program, run away.

• If someone uses scare tactics to vilify an exercise (*Deadlifting WILL BREAK YOUR BACK*), run away.

• If someone is vague, never cites research, and doesn't show any place where they've been peer-reviewed, run away. Vagueness outside of the program is a guarantee that they do not have specifics in their program either.

• If someone publicly shits all over every other type of exercise and program, stay as far away as possible. I love a good Crossfit joke as much as anyone, but if someone is happy doing Crossfit, why would I shit all over that? Hard pass. We can boost our own viewpoints without saying that ours is the only viewpoint.

• If someone shares a ton of great, actionable, researched information, supported by reviews from real people and clear testimonials online, for FREE, that's the program I would buy. Sometimes we think that if they share a ton of info, they don't have anything new to teach us and we can get it all for free from their IG page. Nothing could be further from the truth. If someone has so much information that they can share a ton of great stuff for free, you can be sure they have a ton more where that came from.

Oh yeah, and the women doing great things in S&C? The ones that guy on Instagram couldn't find? Let me help you.

- Mia Lazarewicz at Amplify Fitness (ahem) IG: @thebossiraptor

- Molly Galbraith and Girls Gone Strong IG: @thegirlsgonestrong

- Kelly Matthews IG: @kellylmatthews

- Kaisa Keranin IG: @kaisafit

- Leada Malek IG: @drmalekpt

- Caitlin Hogan IG: @jointjacked

- Saman Munir IG: @sfm_fitness

- Jen Crane IG: @cirque_physio

- Taylor Mei IG: @littletfitness

- Alyssa Olenick IG: @doclyssfitness

- Hayley Madigan IG: @hayleymadiganfitness

There are tons more. These are just a few of my dependables. Use your eyes and your brains to keep a lookout—it's easy to think there's no representation in a space when you aren't looking past the people who are always placed directly in front of you. You start looking? Boom. Right there all along.

All of us, from trainers to doctors to skin care creators, should be collaborating to make the industry better. The general public will only become better educated about themselves if we teach them what they need to know instead of deliberately leaving them in the dark for cash. Health and wellness can be a for-profit industry without conning, misleading, and shaming people into spending their money.

I said in the beginning of this chapter that our main role as health providers is to show people how to care for themselves in the ways in which they struggle the most. Maybe they eat like shit. They see a nutritionist. Maybe they don't ever recognize or handle their feelings. They see a therapist. As trainers, people come to us because exercise is the struggle. So we partner with them to add movement to their life in a way that they can replicate on their own. We don't just show them squats and pushups. *We show them the version of themselves that chooses exercise instead of avoiding it.* Everyone has that side, they just need to see that they like that side of themselves. This change occurs when an exercise habit feels attainable and they feel empowered to attain it. That's what you do as a trainer.

Be better than the hooligans. Better than the influencers posting self-absorbed clownery for clicks. Better than the conference organizers who think that hiring diverse speakers should only be done for quotas. Better than the gym managers who tolerate incompetent, irresponsible trainers because they collect dollars. Bring exercise to the non-exercisers for the one and only reason that you know you can help them enjoy it and benefit from it.

That's how we make the industry better. Although...would I pose looking hot next to pieces of pineapple for a hot pineapple calendar? Yes, I absolutely would. Someone call me about this.

TL; DR

1) The health and fitness industry has enough people who sell scams to unsuspecting buyers. Don't be one of them. Tell people the truth.

2) Decenter your fatphobia. Now.

3) Use a critical eye to evaluate trainers/providers on social media, in person one-on-one, and at conferences. Especially on social media.

4) Social media is NOT the best place to get health information. You need to read real books and study real research. Don't ignore nuance, no matter how captivating the video is.

5) Check your biases about who you want information from. Many people are left out of the front of the industry because they are not masculine white men. Look past them for who else is producing interesting thoughts.

6) Do not attend the SuperDuper Fitness Speaking Conference.

7) Hot Pineapple Calendar is gonna be the name of my wild pop-punk band.

Chapter Twelve: How To Succeed In Service

This chapter is a quickie, designed for anyone who works in a service profession or aspires to work in a service profession. Consider this the summarized handbook you can flip back to when you need advice or a reminder. If you've read the rest of the book, you've already heard me say all these things. But I know there's a Chad out there who will read seven words of this book and then misquote me on Twitter for the next three years, so this is for him.

In no particular order, these are the ways to perform a service job well enough that you'll move up the ladder of whatever profession you're in. And, frankly, non-service jobs as well:

- **Show up for everything you agree to.** Appointments, meetings, work shifts, parties, interviews, lunches, everything. You can say no to stuff, but don't say no to everything. And if you say you're gonna be there, be there. As a business owner and boss, an employee who shows up is like a gift from the gods. It's the number one quality I think of when I want to promote someone. An employee who says no to everything outside regular job parameters is a red flag. An employee who says yes and then doesn't show up? The reddest flag of all.

- **Be prepared.** Be prepared for the personal training session you're about to give, for the meeting notes you're about to take, for the interview you're about to have. Don't show up and ask someone to fill you in on what's happening. Don't decide what you want to do with your client while they're warming up. At the place I used to work, I will never forget seeing another trainer's client come into the gym, ask him if they could do some upper back lifting that day, and seeing the trainer whip out his phone to Google *"upper back exercises."* Do not be this person. Whenever I'm meeting with anyone about accounting, personnel, annual planning, legal, etc, my first question is, "What should I have prepared in advance?" Often the answer is nothing, but you don't want to assume it's nothing.

• **Don't fuck up your schedule.** A long time ago, I made it a personal goal to see if I could go an entire calendar year without fucking up a single session. (Fucking up means forgetting a client, writing down the wrong time, accidentally offering the same time to two people, etc.) At the time I was doing between 1,600 and 1,900 sessions a year. I only succeeded at it one year, but most other years I would only screw up one or two sessions all year. And in spite of my 99.99% success rate, I still felt like absolute shit when it happened. Take people's schedules seriously.

• **Don't offer every time slot under the sun.** To preserve your sanity, set this rule for yourself: you will only offer a time slot to a client if you really want to do a session in that time slot. If it's your lunch break and filling it means you won't eat for nine hours? Don't book that slot unless you're okay with that. If it's a 6AM slot and you have a party the night before? Don't book that slot unless you're okay with that. If it's a Sunday afternoon and the Patriots are playing? Don't book that slot unless you're okay with that. It can be tempting to book every single person for every single time because trainers are so poor for so long and most of us really want to help people get their exercise no matter what. But if it's gonna make you mad or overburdened to have a person in that slot, DON'T FILL IT. You'll do a shitty job in the session and resent the client as if they did something wrong, when you're the one who said yes in the first place. Hold some sanity time for you.

• **Do good work, every time.** Think about your favorite restaurant and your favorite meal that they serve. You go to that restaurant because that meal is delicious every single time. If that meal were only delicious 50% of the time, it wouldn't be long before you found a new restaurant and a new meal where the success rate was higher. I understand that it feels like a lot of pressure, but you need to always put forth the best work that you can, or you will lose your clients. This doesn't mean perfect sessions. It just means good, consistent, thoughtful sessions, where the client can see that you're as invested as they are.

• **Pay attention to the work in front of you.** Get off your phone, mostly, but also stop thinking about your fight with your girlfriend, what you're going to get your mom for her birthday, and how your last session of the day is gonna be a difficult one. You can do those things later. Pay attention to the client you're with right now.

• **Stay educated.** Read everything you can. Be unsatisfied with how little you know. Never, ever assume that you have nothing left to learn. The world these days is packed to the brim with free information. Go find it, retain it, and apply it to be better at your work. Do the same thing tomorrow.

• **Get advice from your coworkers about how they handle their work.** Don't assume that your most experienced coworkers are the only ones with valuable opinions. Just because someone is new to the business doesn't mean they won't have great ideas and a unique perspective. Similarly, just because someone has done a job for a million years doesn't mean they DO have great ideas and a unique perspective. People can burn out, become jaded, or assume they know everything after a long enough period of time. These people won't give you good advice. They'll just talk about themselves and their unhappiness and assume those things apply to you.

• **Ask your clients, coworkers, and bosses about how you're doing at your job.** Especially clients. Are they getting what they want? Have you given them a direction in fitness that they can understand? Are you inadvertently doing stuff they're not particularly interested in or don't enjoy? Sixty minutes isn't very long—you want to make sure that each session has maximum impact. Reassure them that they won't hurt your feelings by giving you feedback. (And then don't let your feelings be hurt. It's not a big deal to be asked to switch gears with someone. I lost a client once because he kept telling me that he didn't want to do high-intensity cardio but I felt it was the most important thing for him to do. After I ignored him many times, he left, and looking back on it, I don't blame him. Remember, it's the client's session, not yours.)

• **Don't cancel people or move sessions or meetings or interviews for your convenience.** People choose workout times for a reason. If you accepted a session, honor the session. If it means sitting at work for three hours where you don't have any clients and you'd rather go home early, big whoop. Pick up a book and study for a while and then see your client at the time they wanted to come in. First of all, your time is not more valuable than theirs. Second of all, it's polite because they've already planned their day around your session, and third of all, there's also a trickle effect. When you take their scheduling seriously, it demonstrates your interest in working with them. When you jerk people's calendars around for no reason, they'll start to think that their session is unimportant to you. And the instant they feel that way, you're going to lose them.

• **But if you can't give a great session, then do cancel it.** Always try to be there. But if you are sick, experiencing personal crisis, distracted by something emotionally heavy, etc, then take care of yourself and don't waste your client's money. Nothing makes me feel worse than when I just do a rote session like a robot, with no thought or care, because I've got something else on my mind and can't get rid of it. Some notable times that I have cancelled clients last-minute: I witnessed a man falling off a roof and exploding on the concrete ten minutes before the session (he survived); I got threatening hate mail at the gym, ransom-note-style; I had to take my mom to the hospital; the city of Boston shut down our gym opening on the day it was supposed to open and I couldn't stop sobbing. I always feel bad when I inconvenience a client, but I would feel worse just giving them random bicep curls and squats because I can't manage anything else. You deserve to care for yourself when you need care, and your clients deserve a provider who can always focus on them when it's their time.

Times when I have not cancelled clients: I have a cold (wear a mask and move on); I have my period (periods fucking suck, but don't get in the habit of cancelling clients once a month for the next thirty years); I had car trouble the night before; I got dumped; I have diarrhea; I have a ton of schoolwork. Figure it out and show up. For the millionth time: service jobs are, for better or worse, in the service of others. You simply can't call out for every reason, even good ones. Get good at compartmentalizing. Handle it after work.

• **Don't talk about your personal life constantly.** A personal training session / massage / facial / etc is a client's time for them. They've made a special point to add you into their busy lives because it's a time for them where no one else can interrupt them. They might love you deeply, but they don't want their hour to be spent listening to you bitch and moan about stuff. They want to bitch and moan about their stuff. I know a few trainers who lost a lot of clients this way. I asked one client why he left his trainer and he said, "He had a lot of problems, and he told me about every single one of them." Woof. This is what I'm talking about in the previous bullet point. That trainer had a lot of personal issues which gave him good reason to miss work often. But at the same time, his clients left him. No one wants to have their session hijacked by their trainer's woes, no matter how valid those woes are.

• **Offer to help.** When someone at the gym needs help, and you are able to give that help, offer it. It's not your client but they're struggling with their bench press? Offer a spot. Someone looks confused about how to adjust the bench? Step in. A member spills their water? Go get a towel. And in general, if you are looking to move up a job ladder, the very fastest way to do it is to see what your boss doesn't know how to do / doesn't do well / doesn't have time for, and offer to do it for them. Then do it well. Watch how quickly you become the favorite.

- **Preserve your reputation when you fuck up.** Your reputation, as Taylor Swift knows well, is the most important currency you've got. All of the above suggestions will preserve your reputation when you're getting things right. But what about when you get things wrong? No one is perfect. I have been late for plenty of sessions, screwed things up, said the wrong thing, injured my clients, overstepped boundaries, broken rules, forgotten clients at six o'clock in the morning, betrayed confidences, shit-talked people within earshot, and sent emails and texts to the wrong recipient (including one where my extremely anxious and exercise-averse 70-year old client proudly told me she had taken a walk that day and I thought it was a text from my friend who just had hip surgery so I texted back, *YES BITCH LET'S FUCKING GOOOOO.* I mean, I was excited my client took a walk too but that would not be my normal professional response lmfaoooooooo) You'll make plenty of mistakes in any job. The way to preserve your reputation in bad conditions is to own the mistake and apologize for it. I don't give a flying fuck if admitting it makes me look like dog shit or costs me or the company money. The value of a genuine, "I'm sorry. I shouldn't have done that," or "I didn't mean to, but it was careless," or "It won't happen again," is priceless. (This is true in your entire life, incidentally. Nothing diffuses a situation faster than a genuine apology, even in really fucked-up situations.)

Practicing these habits will boost you in the best possible way: people will be happy with your work and then talk about you to other people. Your clients will tell their friends about you. Other gym members who don't even train with you will tell their friends about you. Your boss will tell their bosses about you. Your coworkers will notice. If you screw up session times, late-cancel people, or show up unprepared, no one will tell anyone anything about you. And if no one is telling other people about you, you won't be able to make a career in training, or any service at all.

I can hear my readers recoiling at some (or maybe all) of this. Why is every piece of advice about what you can do for other people? What ever happened to self-care? You'll burn out if you're always giving everything away.

A couple thoughts on that, in order of appearance:

First. Service work, when you truly care about the service, is about what you can do for other people. Always. If putting other people first doesn't interest you, I wouldn't recommend personal training as a career. There are other service professions that are less demanding of your time and thoughts, and still other professions that do not require service at all. If you've ever had a mean or unhelpful customer service representative or flight attendant, then you know why a customer-first approach is important.

Next, I am a pro at self-care. Self-care is what allows me to give so much of myself to my work and my people. This is true in all aspects of being a human, not just personal training. I have many hobbies outside of the gym, and those are the places where I can let my brain recharge, do things for me, and be ready for another day of focusing on others.

Finally, you'll only burn out if you are not able to let work be work and let your life outside work be your life outside work. You have to separate them. If I get a flat tire late at night and need to be awake at 5am for my next client, well, tough shit. That flat tire doesn't have anything to do with my work. That's my life outside work. Life outside work is rarely ideal. If you're waiting for ideal life conditions to exist in order to show up at your job consistently, you're gonna be unemployed real fucking fast. I think that's where a lot of people go astray when it comes to work-life balance. They bring their life stress into their work stress, and their work stress into their life stress. No wonder they're exhausted all the time. They never get a break from either one.

Let your work be a break from your life responsibilities. Let your life be a break from your work responsibilities. If both suck, that sucks. But don't let them suck at the same time. Forget about one when you're trying to fix the other. You can only do so much. Just work on fixing one thing at a time instead of trying to fix everything all at once.

A final thought on burnout. Caring for people and being invested in their outcomes doesn't burn me out, it gives me energy. I've been working six-day work weeks since 2009. Two weekend days off when you work in service? It doesn't exist. Holidays? Fat chance. A two-week vacation? Literally never. At my work, there's no lunch break, no texting, no New York Times games, no Instagram, no group chats. At the two-minute junction of one client session with another, I'm often deciding if I want to go pee or eat three bites of food instead. Forty hours of personal training a week is forty full hours, and if you're going to work in the field, you'll need to be okay with that being the bare minimum that you'll be at the gym. Many jobs outside of service do not actually work anywhere close to that. More than a few friends of mine put their salt shaker on their spacebar to keep their laptop logged in at work while they go off and do other things. Remember *Office Space*? "I would say I do about fifteen minutes of real, actual, work per day." That's a lot of jobs, and yes, I'm often jealous of them. But I wouldn't trade with them.

I'm not trying to diminish anyone's job or say that I work harder than other people. I'm just saying that the distractions and escapes that exist in non-service jobs do not exist in personal training/bartending/food service, and that the actual work hours are substantially higher than in many other professions. For me? I don't care. After sixteen years of working like that, I almost never feel burned out. Would I love to have weekends, holidays, and longer vacations? Of course. But not at the expense of losing a job that I love. To me, having the work part of my life be mostly happiness instead of mostly misery is easily worth it. I want this for more people, which is why I wrote this book. If you're still confused about whether you want to make the leap into personal training, let's talk about work for a minute.

I love coaching people on finding work happiness, especially career-changers. Career-changing is so badass!! Someone finally throws up their arms, says, "Fuck this shit," and leaves. That's fantastic. Many more people should do it. And service fields could use more of those highly-motivated, dynamic people in general instead of the "I guess I'll do this because I don't know what else to do" people who typically populate service jobs. Personal training is phenomenally fun work, but it's a pretty bad "stop on the way," if you will. The turnover rate in the field is super high. A lot of people don't know about all the slips, trips, and falls that I've mentioned in this book. They're lost, but think that since they love exercise, they'll just march into a gym and start teaching squats. It doesn't work that way. If you want to work in service but aren't prepared to devote the time and energy it takes to be a trainer, I would recommend choosing a different branch of service, even within the gym itself. My "stop on the way" was a job as a gym equipment cleaner. I got a free membership, worked out a lot, got to know the members, and then had a natural transition into personal training from there. Many of our employees have transitioned from front desk to personal training. It's still not easy, but at least some of the foundation has been set that way. And I may have mentioned this once or twice, but you have to REALLY like working with people. If you're hoping to dive right into personal training simply because you can't find anything else you like, I have another thought.

I don't think that everyone should or even can love their job. There are many unloveable jobs, and someone has to perform them. I suspect that more than a few people who are never satisfied in their work are eternally looking for The One. The One Job that will fulfill them and sustain them as humans and never make them unhappy. Blerg. This is some garbage that we sell hard to kids. Many people won't have—and don't need—emotional engagement with their jobs. It's extremely rare to "find your passion" (I hate that phrase), so quit looking for that. There's nothing wrong with working a job explicitly because it earns you enough money and that's it. You can still derive satisfaction from doing it well. But your work shouldn't feel pointless. It can be boring, or rote, but not pointless. Rote is probably not a reason to make a massive career shift. But pointless absolutely is.

If you're stuck in a pointless job, abandon the idea that you're stuck in it forever because you've already spent so much time there. Recognize the sunk-cost fallacy and GTFO. Otherwise known as the Fuck It, We Ball Principle. Work shouldn't be a demon that you stare down each morning, wondering who will win the wretched battle that day. Life is truly too short for that. You will not get to your deathbed grateful that you stuck it out in a job you hated from day one to day final. You'll be pissed. Work should be more like finding a partner in life. You date a ton of jobs. You look for spark, sure, but what you really look for is ease and compatibility. Are the hard parts torture or are the hard parts fine to deal with? Do you and the job like being around each other with equal vigor or does the job take it all, like a succubus? Just like with humans, there probably isn't The One Job. But also just like with humans, what you really need to know is the Not The Ones. And my experience is that for people who have found Not The Ones in the non-service sector, then service jobs are the answer they've been searching for. People who are suffering at a desk on Wall Street, starving in politics, being devoured by depression in the name of a big tech paycheck, doing mindless spreadsheet work to help someone else earn a lot of money; these people tend to be the ones who realize that they want to use their work time to genuinely help others. These are the people who come to love personal training, physical therapy, nursing, medicine. They hate feeling like work is pointless. They crave the feeling of giving back to others in some way.

If you're still trying to find career happiness, the dream is not to find your passion. The dream is to find a job with negative characteristics that you're willing to live with, because the positive ones outweigh them. It's not romantic, but it's true. Burnout is a phenomenon that comes from a bad partnership. If your work partnership—no matter what work you choose—gives you something back which matches what you put in, you won't struggle with burnout. That could be the money, the atmosphere, the client, or the work itself. If that changes? You also change. No faster way to misery than to stay in a partnership you despise. Be brave, get the fuck out, and get the fuck in to something else. And if that something else is personal training? Awesome! We need you. You might have a client ask you to take off your pants and work in a towel, or a client who doesn't want you to train other men, or a client who says they assume your parents wish you had never been born. But other than that, it's totally great, I promise.

TL;DR

1) This entire chapter was a TL;DR for the rest of the book, so I'm not gonna recap it here except for one thing. If you are deeply unhappy at work, get out of that work. There is a way. Period.

Chapter Thirteen: Final Thoughts

We're finishing up all my rants here, and I hope that you've learned a few things about the behind-the-scenes work of being a personal trainer, the fitness industry, and what a career in service looks like. Personal training is not as easy as people think. Just because you love to lift doesn't mean that's all you need to know about this job. Aside from a love of movement, you need to be a spectacular people person, single-mindedly focused on the person in front of you, and constantly seeking education on your own.

If you remember nothing else from this book, remember these things. Cautionary parts first:

- **Personal training is not about you.** It's not about the workouts you like, the workouts you do, the workouts you'd like to learn, or the workouts you think someone else should be doing. It's not about your convenience, your schedule, or your free time. Personal training is about the client, the workout the client wants to do, the client's convenience, and the client's schedule. Always.

- **You will never know everything.** Everyone who isn't an arrogant dick feels this way about their profession (and, like, life), but it's especially true for health professions. The human body is an area where we have barely broken the surface of its complexity. And even when we understand one human, another may be a total mystery. You will become an expert, but an expert is only defined by the recognition of how much they still do not know. A smart trainer brings in other minds, reads research, searches for the people who might have the information they need.

- **You can't help everyone.** For one, because you don't have time. For two, because not everyone will want your help. Not even if you're the greatest personal trainer in all the land. Just accept this now.

- **You're not the only one who can help someone.** You're not special. The world of healthcare is enormous for a reason. Every person's case is unique and you will not always have the answer. Even when you get the answer, the answer could change. It's why doctors, therapists, auto mechanics, and everyone else has trusted people they ask when they're not sure. If a client is looking for help with something you're not trained in, don't fake it. Ask another trainer, start reading, look around for the education you need to help that client.

- **Do no harm.** People's lives and wellbeing are in your hands. That's not an exaggeration and it's not to be taken lightly. If you're not sure about an exercise being successful, back off. If something looks like it's going wrong, it probably is. Trust your instinct and never be afraid to end a set early, cut out an exercise, or change a workout completely on a dime. You and your client would both rather they stay healthy enough to try again another day.

And now the celebratory parts:

- **Revel in being a teacher.** I stand by this: the reward of teaching is better than any other job. The joy of being able to bring knowledge to someone in a way that improves their life? Are you kidding me? What could be better? All teaching is wonderful, but in personal training, it's a double whammy: they get physical *and* mental education from you.

• **Build your network.** The network of people who train with you and come to your classes is going to become huge. And powerful. Word of mouth is your biggest ally. Put in the effort to earnestly work on and participate in your relationships with people. Do extra work for them that they never see. But don't do it because you want a powerful network. Do it because you're interested in your clients as more than the people who pay your salary. Do it because you want them to succeed and you know you can help them do that.

• **Embrace the unpredictability.** This career is not for the straight and narrow. Your schedule (and pay) will fluctuate every week. Any given session can go spectacularly right or spectacularly wrong, because that's how it goes. Your job is to ride all the waves with your client, no matter how bumpy. Your weekends and holidays will never be yours again, but you won't care. You will always have something new to work on and something new to think about, which is a gift for those of us who crave that.

• **Work on yourself.** You'll learn so much about exercise, mental health, gratitude, the human body, personal relationships, science, communication, and dozens more fields. Use all of that free education to work on yourself. Practice the same things you lecture your clients about, like making changes when things aren't working, or trying new techniques and modalities to supplement your fitness. I recommended meditation and breathwork to lots of clients before recognizing I never did any of it myself. Plenty of trainers get stuck in their own health routines simply because they already know enough about what works. But continuing education applies to you too, not just your clients. Challenge yourself to learn more and be better at your job every day.

• **Be proud of your work right from the start.** Even when you're a new trainer and have limited experience, remember that most people will benefit from exercise immediately, no matter what you do with them. It might be your first training session ever, but you still have the specific and unique opportunity to instantly provide someone with improved health, self-image, and confidence. You can literally contribute to their lifespan. You'll make a difference with every session! You! Will make a difference! With every session! Right from the start! When you look at your work from that perspective, not only will you feel more confident in the service you're providing (even as a beginner), you'll also never mind getting up at 5am. (Well, almost never.)

• **Be joyful.** This is a career for joyful, genuine people. No client wants a sullen, distracted, or disengaged trainer. They want someone who is happy to see them every day, always curious about their body, and deeply involved in the outcomes. And I do not mean that you need to embrace toxic positivity or endless fake cheerfulness. (I hate those people.) I truly believe that when you keep things separate, you can love your work even when you are having a tough time outside of it. I might be crying, furious, or struggling mightily outside of work, and I will nearly always still feel joyful during it.

• **Appreciate humanity.** If ever there were a place to see people as their true selves, it's at the gym. It's the great human equalizer. Everyone is sweaty, smelly, dressed in old clothes, hair a hot mess. They're often rushed for time and grumpy. I've seen A-list celebrities, world-famous academics, internationally best-selling authors, and professional athletes all looking like absolute dog shit. Sometimes they have pee on their shorts or toilet paper stuck to their shoe. Sometimes they forget their clothes at home and have to work out in a button-down, tiny mesh shorts, and dress socks. Often they're revered in the world for one thing or another, and absolutely clueless about fitness. Which is totally fine! It's why personal training exists and why we have jobs. And we trainers often look like shit too; hard not to, when you get up at 4:30am and work in a gym for twelve hours a day. I love stripping the veneer and just letting our bodies be our bodies for an hour or two. This job always reminds me of how much we all have in common with each other. Most of the huge disparities we see in human ideology and human action is part of a boring show. Dropping our guard is refreshing. In real life, when they think no one is watching, people look like trash and fart a lot. Even your heroes. It's great.

In my career, I have had the pleasure of getting blood, spit, sweat, scabs, pubic hair, and yes, semen (thank you, men's steam room) on me at work. I have seen so many testicles and vaginas and accidentally grabbed more than a few boobs and penises. I regularly touch people's sweaty feet and their swassy butts. I've cleaned up finger and toenails that people flick on the floor, and I've had some people with body odor that would decimate the entire population of Boston like a WMD. During my sessions, people have received news of a death, and others have found out that they've been awarded a Nobel Prize. I've held an Oscar award and a client's new baby in the same day.

If this job has given me anything, it's a reverence for the human body and everything it is capable of doing. We are amazing. You are amazing.

The fact that it all mostly works the way it's supposed to is sensational. But we need to give a shit about ourselves if we expect to successfully take our one life from start to finish. That's what you, the personal trainer, do more than anything else. You help people give a shit about themselves. That's beautiful. It's a beautiful career. It's all beautiful. Even those wayward ballsacs.

(Wayward Ballsacs is gonna be the name of my memoir about losing my virginity.)

<u>Acknowledgements</u>

I would first like to thank Eric, who supports me physically and metaphorically, and also makes me pee my pants laughing every minute of the day. What a joy of a person you are. The joyest. Thanks for keeping me around. Of all the things that have been lucky in my life, you're the luckiest thing I ever got.

To Mallory, my brilliant bestie, who agrees that writing is the worst and listens to my daily TED talks about dehydration, existential angst, bad outfits in my closet, and turmeric. Thanks for being down to text ten thousand times a day and inspiring me to wear more lipstick. You're perfect and the way you approach your craft inspires me to be better at mine. I'm so glad we agree that we can both quit writing tomorrow. Not today, but definitely tomorrow.

To JD, my favorite clown, who texts me the most abrasive pep talks in capital letters, long analyses of Taylor Swift songs, and encourages me to ignore all my feelings. Thank you for showing, day after day, what a friend is supposed to be and do. I love how much of our relationship is rooted in false eyelashes. You are fucking amazing.

To Mark, with whom I share equal amounts of poorly-written sentences, cat pictures, and rage about Wordle. The way you live your life is literally a beacon to me. I see what you do and why you choose it and it always makes me want to be better at what I do and choose.

To all my groups: my family, the Pirates, the Dinos, Nu Beta, and the Ninjas. Y'all lift a girl up in every way. Special shout-out to my brother who is annoyingly good at stuff and makes me work super hard just to stay 50% behind him.

To everyone who helped make our gym, Amplify Fitness, a reality, and to everyone who keeps coming back here and kicking ass every day. It's so much fun to watch you making this place what it is.

Most especially, to all my clients. From Whitney, my first client, and carrying through sixteen years of full-time training. Thank you for trusting me with your bodies, for sharing all of the things that you share, for always trying as hard as you can even when the workout is only made up of the worst exercises, and for being my friends. You've taught me everything I know and this book only exists because of you.

Finally, to Batman and Scabby, who sit on my lap any time I'm writing anything. The two most perfect cats ever to exist and I will not be taking questions on this topic.

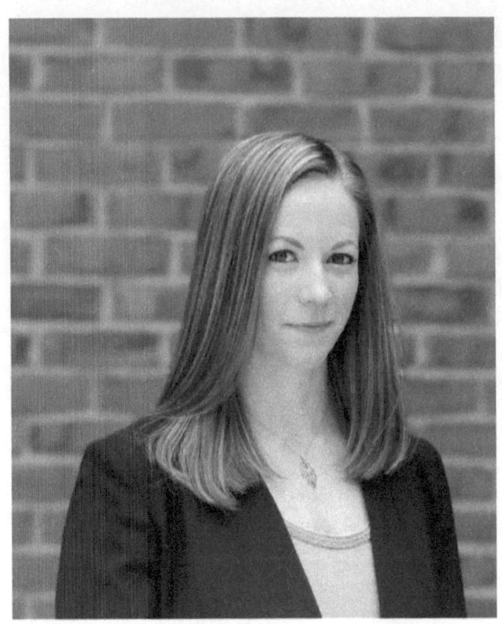

About the Author

Mia Lazarewicz is a certified strength and conditioning coach, fitness writer, lecturer, and American Ninja Warrior from Boston, Massachusetts. Her sharp-eyed training skills quickly made her the most in-demand personal trainer in her company for more than twelve years. Mia is now a co-owner of Amplify Fitness, where she is freer than ever to curse on the gym floor.

Read more at www.trainwithmia.com.